Youth, HIV/AIDS
and Social Transformations in Africa

© **CODESRIA** 2009
Council for the Development of Social Science Research in Africa,
Avenue Cheikh Anta Diop, Angle Canal IV
P.O. Box 3304 Dakar, 18524, Senegal
Website: www.codesria.org

ISBN: 978-2-86978-255-6

Monograph Series

Layout by: Hadijatou Sy
Couver Design: Ibrahima Fofana
Printed by: Graphi plus, Dakar, Sénégal

Distributed in Africa by CODESRIA
Distributed elsewhere by African Books Collective, Oxford, UK.
Website: www.africanbookscollective.com

The Council for the Development of Social Science Research in Africa (CODESRIA) is an independent organisation whose principal objectives are to facilitate research, promote research-based publishing and create multiple forums geared towards the exchange of views and information among African researchers. All these are aimed at reducing the fragmentation of research in the continent through the creation of thematic research networks that cut across linguistic and regional boundaries.

CODESRIA publishes a quarterly journal, *Africa Development*, the longest standing Africa-based social science journal; *Afrika Zamani*, a journal of history; the *African Sociological Review*; the *African Journal of International Affairs*; *Africa Review of Books* and the *Journal of Higher Education in Africa*. The Council also co-publishes the *Africa Media Review*; *Identity, Culture and Politics: An Afro-Asian Dialogue*; *The African Anthropologist* and the *Afro-Arab Selections for Social Sciences*. The results of its research and other activities are also disseminated through its Working Paper Series, Green Book Series, Monograph Series, Book Series, Policy Briefs and the *CODESRIA Bulletin*. Select CODESRIA publications are also accessible online at www.codesria.org.

CODESRIA would like to express its gratitude to the Swedish International Development Cooperation Agency (SIDA/SAREC), the International Development Research Centre (IDRC), the Ford Foundation, the MacArthur Foundation, the Carnegie Corporation, the Norwegian Agency for Development Cooperation (NORAD), the Danish Agency for International Development (DANIDA), the French Ministry of Cooperation, the United Nations Development Programme (UNDP), the Netherlands Ministry of Foreign Affairs, the Rockefeller Foundation, FINIDA, the Canadian International Development Agency (CIDA), IIEP/ADEA, OECD, IFS, OXFAM America, UN/UNICEF, the African Capacity Building Foundation (ACBF) and the Government of Senegal for supporting its research, training and publication programmes.

Youth, HIV/AIDS
and Social Transformations in Africa

Donald Anthony Mwiturubani
Ayalew Gebre
Margarida Paulo
Rekopantswe Mate
Antoine Socpa

Monograph Series

The CODESRIA Monograph Series is published to stimulate debate, comments, and further research on the subjects covered. The series serve as a forum for works based on the findings of original research, which however are too long for academic journals but not long enough to be published as books, and which deserve to be accessible to the research community in Africa and elsewhere. Such works are usually case studies, theoretical debates or both, but they also incorporate significant findings, analyses and critical evaluations of the current literature on the subjects covered.

Table of Contents

Authors

Donald Anthony Mwiturubani
Geography Department, University of Dar es Salaam.

Ayalew Gebre
Department of Sociology and Social Anthropology, Addis Ababa University, Addis Ababa, Ethiopia.

Margarida Paulo
Social Anthropology (MA), Assistant-lecturer/Researcher at University Eduardo Mondlane, Department of Anthropolgy and Archaelogy, Maputo, Mozambica.

Rekopantswe Mate
Sociology Department, University of Zimbabwe, Mount Pleasant, Harare, Zimbabwe.

Antoine Socpa
Anthropologue, Enseignant-chercheur, Université de Yaoundé I, Cameroun.

Preface

The five research reports that constitute this monograph are a fruit of the collaboration between the Council for the Development of Social Science Research in Africa (CODESRIA) and the Social Science Research Council (SSRC) of the USA, two institutions with a longstanding interest in the study of youth and social transformations in Africa. Under the collaboration, 12 young African researchers were able to benefit from fellowships, workshops and the expertise of resource persons, to pursue research on Youth, HIV/AIDS, and Social Transformation.

In Tanzania where high-risk sexual behaviour is common among youths and decreases with increasing levels of education, Anthony Mwiturubani stresses the importance of education for and challenges of accessing and putting HIV/ AIDS related information and skills into practice. He argues that Tanzanian youth, although generally aware of the HIV/AIDS problem and preventive measures, lack a forum in which to express their perceptions and feelings on these issues. The tendency is for adults to impose ideas and decisions on the youth, regardless of the fact that youths and adults have different attitudes, opinions, perceptions and responses to these issues. His study is thus critical of knowledge dissemination practices that do not give youths an opportunity effectively to participate in their design and implementation. He argues for policy makers and planners to understand the context in which youth come to maturity and engage as adults in society.

Gebre focuses on youth in Addis Ababa, mapping how HIV/AIDS prevalence and infection rates appear to decline with age. Primarily and severely affected are the most energetic and productive segments of the population who bear the brunt of the epidemic, a situation which in turn highlights the pivotal role of youth in processes of social transformation. Also discussed is the centrality of heterosexual relations in the transmission of HIV/AIDS, resulting in the proliferation of AIDS orphans. The reality of heterosexual relations is equally at the base of the Ethiopian Government's HIV/AIDS policy, that is geared towards the implementation of preventive programmes and the provision of rehabilitative services for the infected and affected. Within the government's policy framework, Gebre identifies the felt care and support needs of youth living with HIV/AIDS and of AIDS orphans. In addition, he provides a profile of the care and support networks in Addis Ababa, and the challenges that beneficiaries encounter in their attempt to access these services.

Paulo studies the young residents of Mafalala Barrio in Maputo in contribution towards an improved understanding of youth and sexuality in Mozambique, as well as to finding ways of helping HIV/AIDS educational programmes in their intervention endeavours. She calls for a critical rethink of current methods of and assumptions about educational programmes, especially in a context where these very methods and assumptions are failing to curb the rise in HIV/AIDS infections. Paulo points to various socio-cultural factors as key to understanding the perception of sexuality among young people and reason for their ambivalence vis-à-vis messages inviting them to practise 'safe sex'.

On her part, Rekopantswe Mate examines discourses of youth sexuality in rural Zimbabwe from the perspectives of parents, guardians and the youth themselves. She argues that in a bid to be with the world, female youth in Zimbabwe deploy their sexuality and femininity to access modern goods such as biscuits, fizzy drinks, and perfumed lotions, in a context in which they are otherwise marginalised and where these commodities are not accessible. To her, the means by which youth access these commodities constitute a reworking of prevailing local norms of dating and understandings of proper male and female roles leading to social-sexual exchanges between men and women of different ages. The obvious socioeconomic inequalities between the parties limit possibilities of the use of condoms in spite of knowledge about HIV/AIDS. Also, the gendered needs of either party (for men, the quest for sex with young women symbolises virility, spending symbolises economic prowess, and the search for marriageable partners; for women: the need for goods and services accessible with money they do not have and also the search for marriageable partners) seem to make it impossible for safe sex to be practised.

Drawing on his study of Cameroon, Socpa underscores culture as key to understanding the health situation of any community, and as a major influence on the sexual behaviour of individuals and responses towards messages on HIV/AIDS prevention, treatment and care for the infected or affected. He gives a critical overview of the relevance and limitations of cultural explanations of HIV/AIDS, drawing both on existing literature, and on qualitative data based on studies of the Centre and North provinces of Cameroon.

While still very much work in progress, these studies contribute significant empirical data from five different countries to ongoing debates on how youth and social processes in Africa shape and are shaped by the HIV/AIDS pandemic.

Adebayo Olukoshi
Executive Secretary

HIV/AIDS in Tanzania: Knowledge Dissemination Systems and Changing Youth Behaviour

Donald Anthony Mwiturubani

Introduction

The prevention and control of the spread of HIV/AIDS infection remains a priority of many governments, particularly in sub-Saharan Africa, which is estimated to host about 70 percent of the world's HIV/AIDS victims (O'Sullivan 2000; USAID 2001; UNICEF, UNAIDS & WHO, 2002). The prevention efforts regarding HIV/AIDS transmission need to ensure that people, particularly those who are more vulnerable, such as youths,[1] are not exposed to the HIV/AIDS pandemic, and if exposed, have adequate knowledge and skills to prevent infections (Barnett and Whiteside 2002; UNICEF, UNAIDS & WHO, 2002). This needs an approach which provides vulnerable groups such as youths with information and skills, and empowers them to participate in the design and implementation of the programmes that target them (Colling 1998; Shapiro et al., 2003). Two systems of knowledge dissemination exist, namely modern, such as through mass media, and local, such as through stories. For the local methods of knowledge dissemination, the communicator and audience must be present and should speak the same language. On the other hand, in understanding the information and skills provided through modern systems, two aspects are important: one, reliable income for purchasing sources of information, such as radio and newspapers, and second, education for using and understanding the information and skills. Insisting on the role of education in acquiring knowledge about HIV/AIDS through modern systems, UNICEF, UNAIDS & WHO (2002:26) note that:

> Good-quality education fosters analytical thinking and healthy habits. Better educated young people are more likely to acquire the knowledge, confidence and social skills to protect themselves from the virus.

Also studies conducted in Tanzania (Fothal et al., 1996; Kapiga and Lugalla 2002) and elsewhere (Lopez 2002:26; Sigh 2003; UNICEF, UNAIDS & WHO, 2002:27) reveal that high-risk sexual behaviours are common among youths and decrease with increasing levels of education. It follows therefore that education is important for one to access information and skills and put them into practice. Levels of education however have been affected by the socio-economic reforms such as SAPs, which introduced user fees to social services, including education, hence reducing the ability of the youths to access knowledge about HIV/AIDS.

Socio-economic Reforms and the Prevention of HIV/AIDS

The socio-economic trends in sub-Saharan countries indicate that significant number of the population have no access not only to better and quality education but also to formal education in general (Barnett and Whiteside 2002; Lugalla 1995). Since the mid 1980s developing countries and sub-Saharan Africa in particular have undertaken economic and policy reforms initiated by the International Monetary Fund (IMF), the World Bank and other multilateral institutions. Structural Adjustment Programmes (SAPs) that propound free markets and other reforms have affected both positively and negatively the economies of developing countries and peoples' well-being. The introduction of cost sharing in social services, such as education and health, the retrenchment of workers and the removal of agricultural subsidies are some of negative effects of the reforms in these countries. The introduction of school and medical fees, which, for instance, were absent in Tanzania after independence in 1961 under the socialist policies, make it difficult for the majority of the poor Tanzanians to pay for these vital social services. This has increased vulnerability to HIV/AIDS infections in the country since the majority has no access to education and health services. In Tanzania there was an increase in enrolments for primary education in the 1970s in terms of the Universal Primary Education programme (UPE). Every child aged seven was required by law to enrol free for primary education. In the late 1980s and the whole of the 1990s the enrolment rate decreased dramatically (Mbelle and Katabaro 2002; URT 2002b). For instance, between 1993 and 1995 only 45 and 48 percent of eligible males and female children respectively enrolled for primary education (O'Sullivan 2000) with many others dropping out of school due to failure to pay school fees (Lugalla 1995). On average the net enrolment in the 1990s was 54.2 percent and illiteracy rose, with 28.6 percent of the population not able to read and write in any language (URT 2002b:18-19). The trend however reversed after the abolition of fees for primary education in 2000. In 2001, the net enrolment rate reached 65.5 percent (ibid).

In rural areas the removal of agricultural subsidies reduced the ability of the people to pay for education and health services. In Tanzania, there is more illiteracy in rural areas than in urban areas, with higher rates among women (36 percent) than men (20.4 percent) (URT 2002b). Most youths opt to migrate to urban centres to look for jobs. It was estimated, for example, that Dar es Salaam City has been receiving between 20,000 and 50,000 new migrants a year from both rural areas and other urban centres for the last ten years (URT 2003b). Of these, more than 90 percent are youths. At the destination, migrants have limited access to HIV/AIDS and health-related information and health facilities due to a lack of reliable income to pay for the service and purchase sources of information.

Knowledge Dissemination Systems

HIV/AIDS information and skills dissemination has been mainly through modern systems, such as the use of mass media — television, radio, internet, newspapers, and leaflets (Naimani and Bakari 1999; UNICEF 1999; Shapiro et al., 2003; Chatterjee 1999). However, modern knowledge systems are in most cases expensive, particularly when it comes to such sources of information as the internet, radios, televisions and newspapers, which the majority of the population (particularly youths who dominate the unemployed group) cannot afford. Furthermore, they may need someone literate to use them, which marginalise those unable to read or understand the language used (Kinsman et al., 1999; URT 2002b). The modern systems of HIV/AIDS knowledge dissemination hardly take into account the existing socio-economic, cultural, institutional and technological contexts of the audience, and use mainly top-down approaches (Kinsman et al., 1999). This has created conflicts between modern systems of HIV/AIDS knowledge dissemination and socio-cultural standards of the audiences, for instance, in terms of language, content of the programmes, and conduct of the communicators — people delivering information (ibid). This calls for understanding of local knowledge systems employed in disseminating HIV/AIDS knowledge and the way they mediate with modern systems. Local knowledge systems are 'the unique, local knowledge existing within and developed around the specific conditions of women and men indigenous to a particular geographical area' (Grenier 1998:1). These specific conditions of indigenous people include community beliefs, values, skills, attitudes and practices developed over time. Due to conflicts between modern knowledge systems of HIV/AIDS dissemination and socio-cultural standards of the audiences, members of the community may object to the content of the programmes or not absorb the messages at all. Kinsman et al., (1999) observed for instance that parents in Uganda objected when male teachers taught their daughters about

3

condoms, a practice considered to be contrary to their socio-cultural beliefs. In Tanzania, for instance, condom use among youths aged 15-24 years is only 21 and 31 percent for female and male respectively. Furthermore, less than 37 percent of youths aged 15-19 years know the basic three ways (ABC) of avoiding HIV infection — abstinence, be faithful and consistent condom use (URT 2003a). This indicates that either youths do not receive adequate information and skills to protect themselves from HIV/AIDS infections or they do not understand the messages about HIV/AIDS conveyed to them.

Against this background of possible shortcomings of modern systems of knowledge dissemination, the research for this paper proposed to investigate and understand local knowledge systems of HIV/AIDS knowledge dissemination. Furthermore, the study intended to find ways to mediate modern and local systems for designing efficient and effective programmes to disseminate such knowledge. The mediated knowledge dissemination systems need to be gender sensitive and to consider different social groups, such as youths and adults, and their relationship in society (Butler 1990). Mediating modern and local knowledge systems in HIV/AIDS prevention has been proposed elsewhere (Burnnett et al., 1999; Zambia and Myer et al., 2002, South Africa) as a way to improve the acceptability of the information being disseminated. Burnnett et al., (1999) indicate that involving traditional healers in supplying condoms may improve their acceptability and availability, particularly in rural areas. On the other hand, Myer et al., (2002) argue that the lack of access to condoms in South Africa is due to relying on formal health facilities for their distribution. They therefore recommend that the distribution of condoms takes place through both formal and informal systems and that they consider the use of existing social networks.

To understand the knowledge dissemination systems in the prevention of HIV/AIDS and their role in changing youths' behaviour, the following questions were investigated: What are the sources of information about HIV/AIDS for youth in Tanzania? How is the information disseminated (language, time, place, and socio-cultural settings such as gender)? Who disseminates it (adults, youths)? Is the information digestible and accessible to the youths? How do youths perceive and value the methods of information dissemination and information they receive about HIV/AIDS based on modern knowledge systems and local knowledge systems? How do youths organise themselves to understand and prevent the spread of HIV/AIDS among themselves? To what extent has the introduction of education and medical fees affected the dissemination of information about HIV/AIDS?

Methods and Settings

The data for analysis in this paper are from fieldwork conducted in two different geographical locations in Tanzania — one in Kitunda ward in Dar es Salaam City and the other in Burunga ward in Serengeti district, which is located in a rural setting. The choice of these two sites enabled a comparison to be made in HIV/AIDS knowledge dissemination systems and general awareness between urban and rural settings. The intention was also to explore if any similarities and differences existed between urban and rural settings resulting from the process of globalisation. The primary objective of the research was to examine the systems employed in HIV/AIDS knowledge dissemination, and the youths' perceptions, attitudes and responses towards those systems and information received.

The methods employed in data generation included research diaries, semi-structured interviews, focus group discussions, participant observation and document analysis. The research diary method was used for planning and reviewing the day-to-day research proceedings, such as what had been done, problems encountered and what to do next. The method enabled the researcher to find ways to solve problems encountered and hence plan for the next step of the research.

To explore specific issues related to HIV/AIDS knowledge from individual respondents, semi-structured qualitative interviews were conducted. As Flick (1998:76) noted, semi-structured interviews allow respondents to express themselves more openly than in a structured interview, reflecting the respondents' own thinking and feelings. Kitchin and Tate (2000:219) further argue that 'the less structured the interview the greater the flexibility the research has to direct the conversation and to explore specific issues in-depth'. The interview method is one of the effective approaches in health-related studies (Fisher et al., 1996). A total of 35 male youths, 38 female youths, 12 male adults and 10 female adults were interviewed (Table 1). Interviews were conducted at places convenient to respondents, such as vijiwe[2] (mainly for male youths), water collecting points (for females, particularly house-girls), Private Television Show Rooms (for all types of respondents), pubs (for all types of respondents) and ward offices (for adults and a few female youths). Some problems arose in the process of interviewing (Silverman 2001:270). Some respondents did not provide information for fear of a lack of confidentiality concerning the information and the results of the research project. This was the case particularly for male youths found in vijiwe as they feared to be revealed as members. Likewise, house-boys and house-girls feared that the information they provided could be communicated to their employers and that they could lose their jobs. Therefore respondents were assured that information provided would be treated with great confidentiality, and anonymity would be observed. Each participant gave informed and written consent before participating in the research.

Focus group discussions were employed to identify and understand community knowledge, specifically that of youths concerning HIV/AIDS: for example, language, words used, and the feelings, behaviour and attitudes in a particular setting. According to Kitzinger and Barbour (1999:5) a focus group is any group discussion of people provided that the researcher is actively encouraging and attentive to the group interaction. A total of sixteen focus groups were organised — seven in Burunga ward and nine in Kitunda ward. Each group contained five to six participants (Flick, 1998: 118). Focus group discussion is an efficient qualitative data generation technique in that participants tend to provide checks and balances on each other and weed out extreme views. The approach helps to assess how consistent are the views of the participants (Flick 1998:115). Removing those views and statements which are not shared socially increases the validity of the information. Focus group discussions were conducted in the vijiweni, at water collecting points, PTSRs, pubs and ward offices.

Another method employed was participant observation. Though initially this method was not preferred in data generation, it became necessary to adopt it during the fieldwork. To capture some information the researcher had to become one of the members in the private television show rooms (PTSRs) and pubs (Kitchin and Tate 2000). Observation is seeing events as they happen in the natural setting. Marshall and Rossman (1995:79) refer to observation as the systematic recording of events, behaviour and artifacts in a social setting. The method therefore enabled the researcher to understand how the programmes in PTSRs are selected, and to gauge the reaction of the members of different age and gender in the PTSRs and pubs to the programmes.

In addition to the views given during interviews and focus group discussions, document analysis was undertaken. HIV/AIDS policy documents (URT, 2001) and programmes (URT 2002c; 2003a) in Tanzania were analysed. Most programmes designed and implemented prior to 2001 were general, with no specific focus on youths. Most of the programmes treated HIV/AIDS as purely a health problem, and left it to the health sector to design and implement HIV/AIDS programmes.

Results

Sample Characteristics

Details regarding respondents and other participants appear in Tables 1 and 2. The sample comprised youths (73.6 percent) and adults (26.4 percent) (Table 1). Of the youths, 45 and 28.6 percent were male and female respectively, with ages ranging from 15 to 25 years old. Thirty percent of the youths had no formal education or had dropped out of school without completing primary school. The majority of the school drop-outs were domestic servants (house-boys and house-girls), who had migrated to Dar es Salaam to search for jobs after leaving school. The reasons for dropping out of school and not completing primary level education varied among respondents, but the majority cited the failure of their parents or guardians to pay school fees as a major cause. Others mentioned the death of their parents or guardians and the resultant loss of support. A few indicated that they decided to leave schools because for personal reasons, such as poor relationships with their parents, guardians, or teachers. There was no any adult involved in the study with less than primary education level, which indicated that they all benefited from the 1970s Universal Primary Education policy.

As far occupation is concerned, only five percent of youths had employment in the formal sector. Others were either self-employed (poultry keepers, buyers and sellers of eggs, peasants); casual employment (house helps); or day workers. The day worker group represents an unemployed group. In Burunga ward (the rural setting) the main category of occupation is peasant, with a few primary school teachers. A greater variety of occupations was found in the urban setting of Kitunda ward.

Table 1: Gender Distribution of Respondents/Participants (N = 140)

| Location | Youths (N=103) | | | | Adults (N=37) | | | |
| | Male | | Female | | Male | | Female | |
	N	%	N	%	N	%	N	%
Burunga Ward	25	17.9	9	6.4	8	5.7	8	5.7
Kitunda Ward	38	27.1	31	22.1	10	7.2	11	7.9
Total	63	45	40	28.6	18	12.8	19	13.6

Table 2: Socio-economic Characteristics of the Sample

Age (in years)	Youths (N=103) Frequency	Percentage	Adults (N=37) Frequency	Percentage
15 – 17	27	19.3	-	-
18 – 20	31	22.1	-	-
21 – 24	36	25.7	-	-
25 – 30	09	6.4	-	-
30+	-	-	37	26.4
Level of education				
No formal education	13	9.3	-	-
Primary (not completed)	29	20.7	-	-
Primary (completed)	48	34.3	24	17.1
Secondary education	09	6.4	09	6.4
Tertiary education	04	2.9	04	2.9
Occupation				
Poultry keeping	05	3.6	14	10
Peasant	16	11.4	10	7.1
Teacher	07	5	11	7.9
Buying and selling eggs	27	19.3	02	1.4
House servants (house-boys)	10	7.1	-	-
House keepers (house-girls)	11	7.9	-	-
Day works (miscellaneous)	27	19.3	-	-

Knowledge about HIV/AIDS

Generally, youths in Tanzania have some knowledge about HIV/AIDS transmission and prevention methods. There are three main sources from which youths obtain this information. These are, first, the mass media, such as radio, television, internet and newspapers; second, adults (parents, guardians, brothers, sisters, relatives); and third, other youths such as friends, schoolmates, and siblings. The first source here is referred to as the modern method, while the other two are a mixture of both modern and local methods.

Messages about HIV/AIDS

For a message to be delivered three aspects are important: the communicator, the medium and the audience. The communicator is the person delivering the information, also referred to as sources of information under local systems. The medium is the means through which the message reaches the intended beneficiary, also referred to as sources of information under modern systems. The audience is the intended beneficiary of the information.

Communicator

Communicators play an important role in decisions whether to accept or reject a message. When audience attribute the messages to communicators whom they consider credible, the information in the messages is much more likely to prove acceptable, and more attitude change may be expected. But if the audience negatively perceives the character of the communicator, the message will not be properly heard and hence not properly consumed. In Tanzania, under both modern and local knowledge dissemination systems the main communicators of HIV/AIDS messages are young adults and adults. Under local systems alone communicators try to use the language acceptable to the targeted audience. For modern systems linguistic diversity makes this process difficult given the wider audiences targeted. It was observed, for instance, that some people are forced to terminate conversation, switching off the medium, such as radio or television, simply because the communicators' language and characters do not meet the socio-cultural standards of their society. For instance, there is a television commentary where two young adults — a man and a woman — touch each other and a man says 'I love you' a woman replies 'if you love me will you protect me?' The man replies 'why not?', and a woman shows him a condom and says 'if you mean it take this and make it part of our relationship'. While the conversation conveys a clear message on the importance of condoms in HIV/AIDS prevention, the process of delivering it, such as touching and hugging openly between a man and a woman, is against the Tanzanian culture, particularly when the audience comprises both adults and youths.

Medium

The main media for the delivery of messages about HIV/AIDS in Tanzania include television, radio, newspaper, leaflets and one-to-one conversation, such as between friends, parents and children and a presenter and audience at meetings. These sources can be categorised into two major groups based on dissemination systems. The first group consists of modern systems — television, radio, newspaper, leaflets and conversation in conferences. The second group is based on local systems — one-to-one conversation between friends, parents and children, and adults and youths. The one delivering information under local systems may have received it through modern systems.

Peer Educators

Non-governmental organisations (NGOs) have been training peer educators who then educate people, mainly youths, in their residential areas and working places. Peer educators comprise both young men and women. It was clear from the data that the character of peer educators (dress, language and sexual behaviour) influence the messages conveyed to youths. Youths involved in this study reported that they have rejected peer educators because of their misconduct in the process of imparting HIV/AIDS knowledge. Some peer educators have established sexual relationships with youths. Two cases were reported: one a male peer educator who impregnated his fellow female educator before marriage, and another one a male peer educator who impregnated a secondary school girl, for which he was jailed for 30 years.

Feedback Effects

Knowledge is effectively imparted when aided by feedback effects — reactions from the members of the audience to the communicator or to other members of the audience. With respect to modern systems, it was reported that there are no programmes or mechanisms in Tanzania by which members of the audience, particularly youths, can react to the messages delivered. For local systems, there is the opportunity of asking questions, but some youths hesitate to ask for fear that their parents may think that they have already engaged in unsafe sex. However, when female youths are with female adults and male youths with male adults, most youths reported that they felt freer to discuss issues related to sexuality.

Modern Methods of Disseminating HIV/AIDS Knowledge

The main modern methods of disseminating knowledge about HIV/AIDS to the youths and the public in Tanzania are through mass media, such as television, radio and newspapers, and using peer educators who visit people in their residential areas or work places. There are several radio and television programmes and commentaries on HIV/AIDS, which range from prevention methods to caring for the victims of HIV/AIDS. All the youths interviewed and those who participated in focus group discussions indicated that they have heard or watched programmes and commentaries on HIV/AIDS on radio and television. Most of the respondents indicated that they watch television or listen to the radio during the night when they are home. However, out of 103 youths that participated in the research only nine (8.7 percent), all of them living at Kitunda, own televisions, while 30 (29.1 percent) of which only four (3.9 percent) live at

Burunga Ward, own radios. Here, ownership of a television or radio is understood as either family or personal possession. For the adults 16 (43.2 percent), all living at Kitunda, own television and 29 (78.4 percent) own radios, of which eleven (30 percent) live in Burunga ward (Table 3). Although the majority of the rural population (Burunga ward in this case) are too poor to purchase televisions, there is also the problem that the district has no electricity. Given the high price of oil, few can manage to run generators.

Table 3: Possession of Television and Radio
(N = 103 for Youths and 37 for Adults)

Location	Youths				Adults			
	Television		Radio		Television		Radio	
	Freq.	%	Freq.	%	Freq.	%	Freq.	%
Burunga ward	-	-	4	3.9	-	-	11	30
Kitunda ward	9	7.9	26	25.2	16	43.2	18	48.6

Those who do not possess their own televisions or radios watch television and listen to the radio at their friends' homes, private television show rooms (PTSRs, known in Kitunda as Makuti rooms[3]) and in the pubs. The programmes available in PTSRs and pubs are determined by the owner or someone acting on their behalf. For a movie one must pay 50Tshs, equivalent to five US cents, and 100Tshs, equivalent to ten US cents, for watching a football match. Also, one must have the money to get into the PTSR, or to buy a bottle of soda to sit in a pub. Thus, the type of programme determines the number of entrants in the PTSRs and pubs, and hence the amount of money for the television owner. The PTSRs are mainly dominated by youths and they prefer sports, movies and music programmes. The owner of one of the PTSRs in Kitunda indicated that he gets more money when there are football matches. It was clear that there is no great demand for HIV/AIDS programmes in the PTSRs and pubs. However, HIV/AIDS commentaries which precede football and music programmes will be watched by youths in PTSRs and pubs. Watching or listening to HIV/AIDS programmes in the PTSRs or pubs negatively affects the message delivered. The audiences are of different age groups and gender and it is therefore difficult for there to be a common language and practice acceptable to all. For example, it was observed that when a man and a woman participate together to demonstrate the role of condoms in HIV/AIDS prevention, most adults ordered the owner of the medium either to switch it off or change the channel, as they regarded the programme as contrary to their culture.

Youths' Perceptions Towards Modern Methods of Disseminating HIV/AIDS Knowledge

Youths have both positive and negative perceptions on the effectiveness of mass media as a method of disseminating HIV/AIDS knowledge. On the positive side, youths indicated that mass media have enabled them to acquire knowledge about HIV/AIDS prevention methods. Furthermore, mass media as a source of information have enabled youths in Tanzania to understand what is happening elsewhere in the world. However, they indicated that due to economic hardship it is difficult for them to buy the sources and listen to or watch them at their convenience. They also indicated that misconduct or the low reputation of communicators reduced trust in the knowledge delivered. Respondents also state that the youth is on the periphery as far as modern methods of disseminating HIV/AIDS knowledge are concerned. The attitudes and perceptions of the youth are not really incorporated in the programmes.

Local Methods of Disseminating HIV/AIDS Knowledge

Adults over the age of 35 usually are the ones who undertake the role of imparting knowledge to youths, including information on sexuality through story telling. The process of imparting knowledge is gendered, that is, male adults and young adults imparting knowledge to male youths and female elders and adults impart knowledge to female youths. The systems of imparting knowledge are based on taboos, codes of conduct, norms and traditions of the society. For example, adults will draw the moral of their story in such a way as to encourage abstention — mainly for girls; avoidance of idleness; and early marriage for males.

While in urban areas such as Dar es Salaam City individual families are responsible for teaching youth and children, in most rural areas, such as Serengeti district, this task vested in elders and other adults. For instance, in Burunga ward, young men between 15 and 20 years old leave their homesteads and live in a separate place called 'youth villages' with male adults who teach them the societal norms and taboos. On the other hand, female youths remain in their parents' homesteads, living in special local houses where only female adults aged 40 and above are allowed to visit and teach them. They are taught on the dos and don'ts of their society, particularly on the importance of retaining their virginity until they marry. The teaching in the 'youth villages' and special houses takes place twice a year during school holidays.

Apart from these special programmes in the rural areas, elders and adults impart knowledge to their youngsters during the evening when everyone is at home. In urban areas, Dar es Salaam in this case, both men and women may sit together when imparting knowledge. Some youths, especially in Kitunda, indicated that they had had no opportunity to learn from their parents because the latter had died when their children were under ten. In addition, some parents shy away from teaching their children about sexuality, and if they do so, they wait until they are drunk — a situation described by youths as limiting the scope of understanding.

Youths' Perceptions Towards Local Knowledge Systems of Disseminating HIV/AIDS Knowledge

Information about HIV/AIDS disseminated to the youths by adult communicators may have an uncertain reception. Although youths indicated that the system is good as it takes into account the social organisations of society, they try to compare what is taught and what adults actually do in relation to fighting the spread of HIV/AIDS. As one youth commented in one of the focus group discussions at Kitunda:

> adults are telling us to abstain but at the same time they (adults) are having sex with girls of our age group. We are told to listen to adults' words and not to follow their practices.

Such a situation is not likely to make any impact on youths' attitudes and behaviour regarding proper sexual conduct.

Modern Methods of HIV/AIDS Prevention

Youths in Tanzania are aware of the main modern methods of HIV/AIDS prevention, the so-called ABC approach: abstinence, fidelity to one trusted partner, and consistent condom use. Youths indicated however that although not consistently used, condom use is the most common HIV/AIDS prevention method applied. The problem associated with this method however is that one has to buy condoms. Since impoverished youths make up a significant proportion of the unemployed population, some are unable to purchase them.

Local Methods of HIV/AIDS Prevention

The local methods of HIV/AIDS prevention identified are abstinence (mainly insisted on for girls), the avoidance of idleness, and early marriage (mainly insisted for boys) in order to avoid multiple partners. In the rural areas both youths and adults indicated that these are the best methods to prevent HIV/AIDS, but in urban areas youths rejected some of these methods, particularly early marriage, and considered them outdated. However, girls in both Kitunda and Burunga wards indicated that abstinence is the best way of avoiding HIV infection.

13

Youths and HIV/AIDS Programmes and Policies

With the first case of HIV/AIDS reported in 1983 in Kagera region, which borders Uganda (Fothal et al., 1996), and despite the subsequent increase of HIV/AIDS cases, the Tanzanian government was slow in formulating a policy regarding the efforts undertaken to fight the spread of the pandemic, and one only appeared in 2001 (URT 2001). Again, despite the fact that this HIV/AIDS policy contains a special focus on youth, most HIV/AIDS programmes have not involved youth in the design stages. Youths indicated that they are normally asked to participate in implementing programmes designed by adults. This leaves youths — the most vulnerable group[4] — on the periphery of policy formulation.

Discussion

Knowledge Systems and Youths' Changing Behaviour Regarding HIV/AIDS

We have examined two systems of disseminating knowledge about HIV/AIDS in Tanzania — modern and local knowledge systems. The analysis of these systems based on the data obtained from the field, and from published and unpublished works, indicates that none of them is very effective by itself in imparting HIV/AIDS knowledge to Tanzanians, particularly to the high-risk group of population such as youths. Youths trust neither the people delivering information nor messages delivered. One of the main reasons given was that youths are not involved in designing the programmes to disseminate HIV/AIDS information, which thus hardly take into account the needs of youths. Although a study conducted in Tanzania (UNICEF 1999) shows that all Tanzanian media — television, radio, newspapers — include stories and commentaries on HIV/AIDS, the change of behaviour among the vulnerable population has been insignificant. Few are ready either to abstain or use condoms consistently.

The findings from this study indicate that youths are aware of the ways in which knowledge about HIV/AIDS is disseminated, and they are aware of methods employed in preventing infection. This finding is contrary to that in one study that concluded that less than 37 percent of youths in Tanzania know the three ways of avoiding HIV infection — abstention, fidelity to one partner, and consistent and correct condom use (URT 2003a). However, illiteracy and the lack of income to purchase the sources of information have negatively affected HIV/AIDS knowledge dissemination, particularly through modern systems. This is among the effects of structural adjustment programmes (SAPs), which introduced user fees in social services such as education. Adults also seem to be an obstacle for youths to receive HIV/AIDS information from modern systems. Since adults possess the medium in which information is disseminated, they tend to select the programmes to be watched without regard to the youths' needs or wishes. Adults prefer programmes in a specific language, and may switch off programmes in other languages regardless of whether the language is appropriate to youths or not. Local systems could be the most effective, but many urban youths do not trust them either. They argue that their elders do not have up-to-date and adequate information. However, in the rural areas local systems seem to be effective.

Gender Roles in Knowledge Dissemination

Given gender differences in responsibility for both reproductive and productive tasks the possibility of gender-based differences in vulnerabilities to HIV/AIDS might be expected. The gender-based differences in HIV/AIDS infections can be explained in several contexts. Among these are the existing socio-cultural settings in African societies and the differences in accessing knowledge about HIV/AIDS. The findings reveal for instance that in Tanzania there is more illiteracy among women than men and that awareness about condom use is lower among female youths as compared to male youths. A study conducted in Tanzania (URT 2003a) reveals that about 50 percent of admissions in hospitals due to abortion-related complications are comprised of youths aged between 15 and 24, which indicates that youths are practising unsafe sex.

Most programmes and commentaries on HIV/AIDS prevention in the media in Tanzania have placed much emphasis on the roles of girls in either resisting the sexual advances of men or insisting on the use of condoms. However, youths, both male and female, indicate that girls have less power in making decisions on the use of condoms. They further argue that girls have been insisting on the use of condoms mainly to prevent pregnancies. Despite the prominent role of female youths in HIV/AIDS prevention, there are no specific programmes to disseminate knowledge that target or involve them from the first stage of programme design. Instead youths, especially female, are portrayed as weak and unable to make an appropriate contribution in the decision making process. It is therefore important for communicators to involve actively youths in programme design and give both males and females equal roles in insisting on abstinence and practising safe sex. Such programme designs need to include both modern and local systems in order to cater for socio-cultural issues which might affect the acceptance of the programmes.

The Interface Between Modern and Local Knowledge Dissemination Systems

Both modern and local knowledge systems have significant contemporary roles to play in HIV/AIDS knowledge dissemination in Tanzania, particularly to youths. Already there are links between these systems, as some adults communicators report that they receive information through modern systems and impart them to the youths in local fashion. The National Policy on HIV/AIDS in Tanzania also incorporates the need to link modern and local systems: 'Customary practices and cultural institutions that provide opportunities for public awareness shall be utilised' (URT 2001:17).

However, the mechanisms to mediate the two systems are not yet clear. There is therefore a need to develop a common set of definitions, a common language, and common content for programmes to so that they are adapted to both modern and local knowledge systems. To achieve this aim, programme designers from both systems should sit together and define socio-cultural parameters to be included in HIV/AIDS knowledge dissemination programmes. There should be consensus between members representing each system. Members in each group should be from different social backgrounds, such as young men and women. This calls for a bottom-up participation approach.

Conclusion

This paper demonstrates that majority of the youths in Tanzania know of the problem of HIV/AIDS, including the preventive measures. What they do not know is how to address the problem properly. Youths lack a forum in which to express their perceptions and feelings. They only give opinions on the ideas imposed by adults and have little power to influence any decision. The methods employed in HIV/AIDS knowledge dissemination, whether based on modern or local approaches, do not give youths an opportunity effectively to participate in their design and implementation. However, it is clear that youths and adults have different attitudes, opinions, perceptions and responses to these programmes, which make it necessary for both groups to be involved. The participation of the youth in these programmes has however been undermined by widespread illiteracy, which is mostly a function of the introduction of school fees during the implementation of structural adjustment policies after a period when primary education had been a free service in Tanzania. Employing local systems, and utilising local languages, can reduce the problem of illiteracy. There is, therefore, a need for policy makers and planners in different social development projects including those against HIV/AIDS to understand the context in which groups such as the youth come to maturity and engage as adults in society.

Acknowledgements

The research for this paper was assisted by the Social Science Research Council (SSRC) New York and the American Council of Learned Societies, Africa Regional Advisory Panel in partnership with the Council for the Development of Social Science Research in Africa (CODESRIA), and the South African National Research Foundation's Africa Youth and Globalisation Fellowship. We are grateful to these institutions. We are also grateful to the University of Dar es Salaam for providing us with research clearance to conduct fieldwork. We further thank Dar es Salaam and Mara Regional Secretaries, Ilala and Serengeti District Secretaries and Burunga and Kitunda ward Executive officers for granting us permission to conduct research in their respective administrative areas. Finally, we are grateful to youths and adults who volunteered to participate in our research.

Notes

1. 'Youth' in this paper refers to people aged between 15 and 25.
2. Vijiwe are places where people, particularly youths, meet for informal discussion. Adults and government leaders regard these places as sources of criminal conduct, particularly for petty drug trafficking.
3. PTSRs are called Makuti rooms because they are constructed using coconut tree leaves — makuti in Swahili.
4. In 2002 it was estimated that over two million people (about 5.9 percent of the total population) were living with HIV/AIDS in Tanzania, of which 15.2 percent were youths aged 15 to 24, and 70.5 percent were young adults aged between 25 and 49 (URT, 2001; 2002a). Among the new infections, 69 percent are in the 15-24 age bracket with slightly more than half of these among girls (URT, 2003).

References

Barnett, T. and Whiteside, A., 2002, *AIDS in the Twenty-First Century: Disease and Globalisation*, New York, Palgrave Macmillan.

Burnnett, A., Baggaley, R., Ndovi-MacMillan, M., Sulwe, J., Hang'omba, B., and Bennett, J., 1999, 'Caring for People with HIV in Zambia: Are Traditional Healers and Formal Health Workers Willing to Work Together?', *AIDS CARE*, Vol. 11, No. 4, pp. 481-491.

Butler, J., 1990, *Gender Trouble: Feminism and the Subversion of Identity*, London, Routledge.

Chatterjee, N., 1999, 'AIDS-related information exposure in the Mass Media and Discussion within Social Networks among Married Women in Bombay, India', *AIDS CARE*, Vol. 11, No. 4, pp. 443-446.

Colling, J. A., 1998, 'Children Living in a World of AIDS: Guidelines for Children's Participation in HIV/AIDS programmes', *A Children and AIDS International NGO Network* (CAINN) Publication.

Grenier, L., 1998, *Working with Indigenous Knowledge: A Guide for Researchers*, Ottawa, IDRC.

Fisher, G., Pappas, G., and Limb, M., 1996, 'Prospects, Problems and Pre-requisites for National Health Examination Surveys in Developing Countries', *Social Science and Medicine*, Vol. 42, No. 12, pp. 1639-1650.

Flick, U., 1998, *An Introduction to Qualitative Research*, London, Sage Publications.

Fothal, D., Mdhalu, F. S., and Dahoma, A., 1996, 'AIDS in Tanzania', II International Conference on AIDS, Paris, Abstract No. S17F.

Kapiga, S. H., and Lugalla, J. L. P., 2002, 'Sexual Behaviour Patterns and Condom Use in Tanzania: Results from the 1996 Demographic and Health Surveys', *AIDS CARE*, Vol. 14, No. 4, pp. 455-469.

Kinsman, J., Harrison, S., Kengeya-Kayondo, J., Kangesigye, E., Musoke, S., and Whitworth, J., 1999, 'Implementation of a Comprehensive AIDS Education Programme for Schools in Masaka District, Uganda', *AIDS CARE*, Vol. 11, No. 5, pp. 591-601.

Kitchin, R. and Tate, N. J., 2000, *Conducting Research into Human Geography, Theory, Methodology and Practice*, England, Pearson Education Limited.

Kitzinger, J. and Barbour, R. S., 1999, 'Introduction: The Challenge and Promise of Focus Groups', in Barbour, R. S. and Kitzinger, J., eds., *Developing Focus Group Research, Politics, Theory and Practice*, London, Sage Publications, pp. 1-20.

Lopez, V. M., 2002, 'HIV/AIDS and Young People', Consultant Report, New York.

Lugalla, J., 1995, 'The Impact of Structural Adjustment Policies on Women's and Children's health in Tanzania', *Review of African Political Economy*, No. 63, pp. 43-53.

Marshall, C., and Rossman, G. B., 1995, *Designing Qualitative Research*, 2nd edition, London, Sage Publications.

Mbelle, A. V. Y., and Katabaro, J., 2002, 'School Enrolment, Performance, Gender and Poverty (Access to Education) in Tanzania Mainland', Final Report Submitted to Research and Poverty Alleviation (REPOA), Dar es Salaam.

Myer, L., Mathews, C., and Little, F., 2002, 'Improving the Accessibility of Condoms in South Africa: the Role of Informal Distribution', *AIDS CARE*, Vol. 14, No. 6, pp. 773-778.

Naimani, G. M. and Bakari, V., 1999, 'Contribution of Radio Drama "Twende na Wakati" on Family Planning and HIV/AIDS Awareness in Tanzania', UPSD.

O'Sullivan, P., 2000, *HIV/AIDS in Sub-Saharan Africa: A Development Issue for Irish Aid*, Dublin.

Shapiro, D., Meekers, D., and Tambashe, B., 2003, 'Exposure to the "SIDA dans la Cite" AIDS prevention Television Series in Côte d'Ivoire, Sexual Risk Behaviour and Condom Use', *AIDS CARE*, Vol. 15, No. 3, pp. 303-314.

Sigh, S., 2003, 'Study of the Effect of Information, Motivation and Behavioural Skills (IMB) Intervention in Changing AIDS Risk Behaviour in Female University Students', *AIDS CARE*, Vol. 15, No. 1, pp. 71-76.

Silverman, D., 2001, *Interpreting Qualitative Data, Method for Analysing Talk, Text and Interaction*, 2nd edition, London, Sage Publications.

UNICEF, 1999, 'Children in Need of Special Protection Measures: Summary Report', Dar es Salaam.

UNICEF, UNAIDS & WHO, 2002, *Young People and HIV/AIDS: Opportunities in Crisis*, New York.

United Republic of Tanzania (URT), 2001, *National Policy on HIV/AIDS*, Prime Minister's Office, Dodoma.

URT, 2002a, 'Epidemiological Fact Sheets on HIV/AIDS and Sexually Transmitted Infections', UNAIDS, WHO, Dar es Salaam.

URT, 2002b, *Poverty and Human Development Report*, Dar es Salaam, Mkuki na Nyota Publishers.

URT, 2002c, *National AIDS Control Programme (NACP)*, Dar es Salaam, Ministry of Health.

URT, 2003a, 'Draft for Preparing an Operational Plan for the Health Sector Response on Young People and HIV/AIDS', Dar es Salaam, Ministry of Health.

URT, 2003b, 2002, *Population and Housing Census*. General Report, Dar es Salaam.

U.S. Agency for International Development (USAID), 2001, 'Press Release No. 097', Available at http//www.usaid.gov.

HIV/AIDS in Addis Ababa: Understanding the Care and Support Needs and Problems of Young People Living with HIV/AIDS and of AIDS Orphans

Ayalew Gebre

Introduction

It is common knowledge that the HIV/AIDS prevalence rate in Ethiopia is already one of the highest in the world. According to the latest statistics provided by the Disease Prevention and Control Department of the Ministry of Health (2002), 2,2 million persons (6.6 percent of the entire population) currently live with the HIV virus. Two hundred thousand of these HIV cases are reported to be children. The same source projects that the rate of prevalence will remain generally consistent until 2010. Accordingly, the prevalence rate will rise to 2.6 million in 2006 and 2,9 million in 2010, which figure involves both people living with the virus and full-blown AIDS cases.

The above study, with data drawn from 34 sentinel surveillance sites around the country, reported an average urban prevalence rate of 13.2 percent. The current prevalence rate for Addis Ababa is 15.6 percent, after five other urban centres of the 34 sentinel sites. The period from 1989 to 1995 marked a steep increase in HIV prevalence for Addis Ababa. However, a gradual decline in prevalence rates started in 1995 and continued to date. Given sustained prevention and control efforts, the projection for the coming years is that there will still be a further let up in the prevalence rate for the capital, with prospects of increased decline.

The study also furnishes a set of findings on age and sex specific rates of HIV prevalence for the country. Thus, it indicates the peak ages of AIDS cases to be 25 to 29 for both females and males. Taking into account eight years of the incubation period, on average, between infection and the emergence of the full-blown disease, the mean ages in which people get infected range from 15 to 24 for females, and 25 to 34 for males. According to available data, by far the largest numbers of people infected with HIV are concentrated in the age groups of 15 to 24, and slightly to a lesser extent, 25 to 34 for females. The age groups of 20 to 24 and 25 to 29 represent the highest rates of infections for males. The variations in the sex and age distribution of the HIV cases may be explained by early sexual activity among young girls and the fact that they often have older partners. The thrust of the findings is that prevalence and infection rates appear to be declining with age.

The evidence reinforces the implications of the current prevalence statistics that are obviously serious and far-reaching. Primarily and severely affected are the most energetic and productive segments of the population who bear the brunt of the epidemic. The theme 'Young People: Force for Change', chosen for the 1998 World AIDS Campaign, was no doubt prompted by the realisation and appreciation of these facts. The campaign brought to the fore the power of the young in the process of introducing and implementing changes. It emphasised that the future of the epidemic lies in their hands. The life styles that they adopt today can determine which course the epidemic is going to take over the years to come. Research has amply shown that the young will adopt safer sexual behaviour provided that they are given the necessary information, means and skills around HIV/AIDS prevention and control, including care and support for the infected and affected. Increased orphan-hood is a single major dimension of the impact exerted by HIV/AIDS. Men and women dying from HIV/AIDS-related causes in their prime child rearing ages often leave orphans behind them. In this context, an AIDS orphan is someone under 15 who has lost a mother to AIDS. However, given the important role heterosexual relations play in the transmission of the virus, a child is most likely to lose both parents to the disease although the deaths may occur at different time intervals. The recent study by the Disease Prevention and Control Department of the Ministry of Health (2002) projects that the number of AIDS orphans in Ethiopia, which was 1,2 million in 2001, will jump to 1,8 million in 2007 and to 2,5 million in 2014. The Addis Ababa City Government Health Bureau (AACGHB 2000) and the Organisation for Social Services for AIDS (OSSA, 2000) provide two different figures on AIDS orphans in the city. The former puts the number at 20,000 and the latter at 30,000 for the year 2000, during which year each organisation conducted the study. Both studies projected that the number would increase to 64,000 in 2004 and 145,000 in 2014 (AACGHB 2000; OSSA 2000).

The Ethiopian Government issued a national policy on HIV/AIDS in 1998. The policy aims to direct the various efforts put forth to mitigate the impact of the pandemic. To this end, two government bodies have been set up with different but complementary mandates and responsibilities. The government has vested in the Disease Prevention and Control Department (DPCD) of the Ministry of

Health (MoH) the responsibility for the planning and implementation of HIV/ AIDS prevention and control programmes. It has also established an HIV/AIDS Prevention and Control Office (HAPCO), which is responsible for mobilising multi-sectoral and grass root efforts in the fight against the epidemic. The national policy on HIV/AIDS carries two broad components. It is geared towards the implementation of preventive programmes and the provision of rehabilitative services for the infected and affected. The care and support system lies at the heart of the rehabilitative component of the policy. In fact, one of the stated policy objectives relevant to this study runs in these words: 'Make the necessary provision of care and support to people living with HIV/AIDS and their affected family members'. Within this policy framework, this study endeavours to identify the felt care and support needs of young people living with HIV/AIDS (PLWHA) and AIDS orphans in Addis Ababa. In addition, it provides a profile of the care and support networks currently in place in the city, and the challenges that beneficiaries encounter in their attempt to access the services.

Research Objectives

This research aimed to achieve the following objectives:

(i)   Ascertain the needs and problems of young people living with HIV/AIDS and AIDS orphans, from their own point of view;

(ii)   Establish how these young people prioritise these needs and problems along gender lines, among other factors.

(ii)   Evaluate the effectiveness of these networks in the light of the judgment and perception of beneficiaries.

(iv)   Find out the challenges encountered in the process of accessing available care and support services.

(v)   Obtain community feedback from selected research populations on the practical remedies towards the improvement and expansion of existing care support services.

Research Methods

The research methodologies employed involve four participatory techniques of qualitative data collection:

(i)   Key informant interviews: Concerned and selected community members such as the elderly, community leaders, teachers, students, health workers, and leaders of youth associations and anti-AIDS clubs were interviewed with a view to drawing up a general community perspective on the most pertinent themes of the study. Major questions presented to key informants using this method had to do with the social impact of HIV/AIDS, stigma issues and social support systems.

(ii) Focus group discussions: Discussions were held with male and female burial associations (Iddir) leaders, Woreda (district) HIV/AIDS council members, and young people living with HIV/AIDS who are members of Dawn of Hope and Mekdim Ethiopia, Associations of PLWHA. The purpose of the discussions was to generate the required data on the needs and problems of the affected community members, and the services provided to address them.

(iii) Individual in-depth interviews: Young people living with HIV/AIDS (male and female) and AIDS orphans were interviewed on person-to-person basis, so that they would express their experiences with HIV/AIDS, recount the community reactions to their status, inform us of their coping mechanisms, as well as their concerns, hopes, and life styles.

(iv) Participant observation: This method was employed in a more restricted sense of the term, to gather information through an intensive face-to-face interaction with the subjects of the study. Participant observation tends to be a more active process than direct observation. It involves prolonged contact and frequent encounters, particularly with informants having 'specialised' knowledge about matters under investigation and who display the goodwill to share experiences with the investigator. The researcher pursued participant observation as an ideal method of personal involvement and interaction to make the best possible use of opportune social situations.

Description and Analysis of Field Data

Needs and Problems of Young PLWHA

In-depth interviews and focus group discussions took place separately with young males and females living with HIV/AIDS, who are members of the Dawn of Hope and Mekdim Ethiopia Associations of PLWHA. The purpose was to identify the felt needs and problems of young PLWHA in Addis Ababa in connection with the existing care and support institutions and access to the services they provide.

The major category of need as prioritised by the informants is health care, in the physical, economic and psychological senses.

With regards to health care, the following needs have been identified as requiring close attention:

(i) Access to standard and comprehensive medical services;

(ii) Urgent treatment of opportunistic infections and AIDS-related illness prior to the person becoming susceptible to their weakening effects;

(iii) Regular and continuing medical check-ups by health professionals;

(iv) Cessation of the practice of denying hospital beds to AIDS patients on the grounds that they are terminally ill and there is no cure for the disease. Instead as many hospital beds as are affordable should be reserved for them;

(v) Establishment of a specialised HIV/AIDS hospital where young PLWHA and AIDS patients can easily access the type of medical service they need;

(vi) The provision of home-based nursing and medical treatment to bed-ridden patients with full-blown AIDS;

(vii) Access to anti-retroviral treatment with the administration of the necessary medical procedures.

Physical needs have been prioritised as the second most important. These include nutrition, decent housing, and sufficient clothing. AIDS is known to have debilitating effects on the patient by undermining his or her immune system. Thus, regular and adequate nutritional supplies are a major requirement to enable the patients to withstand opportunistic infections and thereby promote their health. Besides, AIDS patients need a good amount of rest in a home environment free of worry and anxiety to the extent possible. To meet this need, provision of decent housing with modest furnishings is vitally important. As their health deteriorates, patients are confined to the home, in which case they will need adequate and cleaner quantities of bedding. Moreover, sufficient supplies of detergents, cleansers, and insect repellants will be necessary to keep things in a good sanitary condition and prevent further infections.

In the third place, interview and discussion participants have described socio-economic needs of young PLWHA as deserving the maximum possible attention of care and support agencies. Bed-ridden and debilitated patients especially need financial support to deal with day-to-day cares and problems. Others living with the virus but still able to work and fend for themselves also need to be supported financially so that they can be rehabilitated as productive and self-supporting members of the community. Those forced to move to other areas under the pressures of stigma and discrimination by family members, neighbours, and peers seek financial backing to pay house rents among other necessities. They also need support to cover expenses incurred for social activities as well as the payment of school fees, supplies of educational material and uniforms for themselves or their children. Another great social need stated is free and unhindered access to social participation in institutions and events such as burial, women, and youth associations, socio-religious gatherings, wedding and other festivities.

Young PLWHA also have strong psychological needs that they want considered as part of the care and support service. They desire to be shown proper and genuine empathy and affection, which, if they are sure they are given, will strengthen their will to live and their powers to resist the impact of the illness. They feel that they need access to participation in all social activities and events without discrimination. Further, access to regular and continuing counselling services, both home-based and institutional, is very desirable. Finally, there is the need for provision of care and support by family members, neighbours, and home-based care agents in the form of nursing, consistent dietary follow-up, protection against communicable infections, timely delivery to health institution when necessary, supply of adequate information concerning responsible sexual behaviour, and support for regular habits of physical exercise.

Currently Operational Care and Support Programmes

An inventory was drawn up of HIV/AIDS and orphan care and support institutions in Addis Ababa (government, NGOs and CBOs) in order identify the type and coverage of the services provided. Tables 1 and 2 give details the existing care and support institutions for orphans and for PLWHA by type of service provided.

Focus group discussions were conducted on this subject exclusively with young PLWHA who are members of Dawn of Hope and Mekdim Ethiopia associations of people living with HIV/AIDS. Their responses show that currently the bulk of care and support services for PLWHA is being rendered by these two associations, which are so far the only ones of their kind in the country.

HIVAIDS counselling is the single most important service given. The participants in the discussions reported that they have all been receiving regular counselling services on individual and group bases. 'Professional counselling enables us cope successfully with the effects of the virus and the resulting social stigma', they claimed. In fact, a great number attributed their ability to survive longer directly to the counselling that they received. They added, 'counselling imparts the solace and vigour that one truly needs to accept the reality of living

Table 1 : AIDS Orphans Care and Support Institutions

No.	Name of Organisation	Type of Service Provided
1.	Aba Woldethensaye Gizaw Mathers & Children Welfare Association	Medical, Financial and Educational Support.
2.	Abebech Gobena Orphan Project	Medical, Nutritional and Educational Support.
3.	Birhane Hiwot Children's Village & Family Services Organisation	Medical, Financial and Educational Support
4.	CCF-Edget Ber Area Project	Medical, Financial, Material, and Educational Support.
5.	Community Based Integrated Sustainable Development Organisation (CBISDO)	Medical, Nutritional, and Clothing.
6.	Enat HIV orphan project	Medical, Nutritional, Educational, and Housing
7.	Hiwot HIV/AIDS Prevention, Care & Support Organisation.	Financial, Educational, Clothing, and Skill Training.
8.	St. Mary's Orphan Support Program of the Daughters of Charity of the Ethiopian Catholic Church.	Nutritional, Educational, Housing, Clothing, Psychological Sup.
9	Hiwot Ethiopia	Financial, Material, and Legal Support
10.	Yehiwot Tesfa (Counseling and Social Service Centre of the Ethiopian Evangelical Church of Mekane Yesus)	Nutritional, Educational, Housing, Clothing, Psychological Sup. Medical, Educational, Clothing, Counselling, Recreational
11.	Hope for Children	Medical, Financial, Nutritional, Educational, Clothing,
12.	Mary Joy Aid Through Development	Recreational, and Social Support
13.	Medhin Social Centre	Financial, Nutritional, Material, Educational, and Clothing.
14.	Medical Missionaries of Mary-MMM (Counselling and Social Service Centre (CSSC)	Medical, Nutritional, Material, Educational, Clothing, Shelter, and Psycho-Social
15.	Organisation of Social Service for AIDS (OSSA)	Financial, Nutritional, Educational, and Counselling
16.	Pro Pride	Educational, and Counselling
17.	Selame Children's Village	Medical, Nutritional, Educational, Clothing, and Housing
18.	Children AID Ethiopia (SHAD-ET)	Medical, Nutritional, Educational, and Skill Training
19.	Dawn of Hope-Ethiopia	Medical, Material, Educational, Home-Based Care
20.	Mekdim Ethiopia	Medical, Financial, Nutritional, Educational, Clothing, Shelter, and Home-Based Care
21	Woreda HIV/AIDS Council	Financial (School Fee), Nutritional, Educational, Shelter, Clothing, and Home-Based Care
22	Burial Associations (*Iddir*)	Nutritional, Educational, and Clothing.

27

Table 2: Young PLWHA Care and Support Institutions

Name of Organisation	Type of Service Provided
Medical Missionaries of Mary (MMM)	Nutritional, Financial, Skill Training
Organisation of Social Service for AIDS (OSSA)	Nutritional, Financial, Skill Training
Pro Pride	Nutritional, Financial, Religious, Micro-Credit Facility
Medhin Social Centre	Financial, Nutritional, Material, Educational, and Clothing
Mary Joy Aid Through Development	Medical, Nutritional, and Religious
Hiwot HIV/AIDS Prevention, Care and Support Organisation	Medical, Nutritional, Financial, and Educational
Community Based Integrated Sustainable Development Organisation (CBISDO)	Medical, Nutritional, Shelter, and Educational
Aba Woldethensaye Gizaw Mothers & Children Welfare Association	Medical, Shelter, and Educational
Children AID Ethiopia	Medical, Nutritional, Material, Financial, Shelter, Micro-Credit Facility
Dawn of Hope Ethiopia	Medical, Nutritional, Material, Legal, and Home-Based Care
Mekdim Ethiopia	Medical, Nutritional, Legal, Shelter, and Home-Based
Woreda HIV/AIDS	Financial, Nutritional, Educational, Shelter, Clothing, Home-Based
Burial Associations (Iddir)	Nutritional, Educational, and Clothing

with the virus and facing up to the challenges it involves'. Therefore, they continued, 'we have been able not only to live longer but also feel better and stay healthier'. Different forms of socio-economic support are another type of service available. Young association members under family care receive Birr 75 per head monthly and those living on their own Birr 150 per head monthly, to help them cover their living expenses. Up to Birr 400 is provided to members undergoing medical treatment to assist them to buy medicine on prescriptions.

Home-based care is a third principal type of care and support service rendered by the associations of PLWHA. It is given to bed-ridden patients and children living with the virus. Trained home care agents, who may themselves be living with the virus provide the service. The involvement of PLWHA in the provision of home-based care has a dual advantage. Besides creating job opportunities, it enables them show in practical terms love and compassion to others under like circumstances. Young PLWHA who served as home-based care agents expressed their thoughts and sentiments as follows:

> Providing home-based care satisfies us the most. Patients feel psychologically restored and empowered when given services accompanied with expressions of commitment, personal interest in them and reassuring words. When they feel healthy and strong enough to do some work, they feel motivated to serve as home-based care agents themselves.

NGOs are the second important institutions implementing care and support programmes in Addis Ababa, next to the associations of PLWHA. Voluntary counselling and testing services (VCT) is a major form of HIV/AIDS care and support provided by NGOs. VCT service enables individuals to obtain personal information they need regarding the modes of HIV/AIDS transmission and the methods of prevention. In the case of infected persons, it provides the necessary psychosocial support to withstand the stress resulting from the knowledge of sero-status. It encourages HIV positive individuals to value life and their relationships with others. Thus, they helped to develop or maintain an optimistic view of life, place things in a realistic perspective and assure themselves that they are still needed regardless of their status. Hence, the VCT service makes up a vital component of HIV/AIDS care and support systems as an effective strategy of control and prevention. The institutions identified by young PLWHA and community members as actively perusing the provision of VCT are Mary Joy Aid through Development, Medical Missionary of Mary Counselling and Social Service Centre (MMM), Hiwot Tesfa, Organisation for Social Service for AIDS (OSSA), and CARE Ethiopia.

In addition to VCT, NGOs are also involved in the distribution of material and nutritional supplies to the PLWHA. These include the donation of grains, cooking oil, clothing, and cash.

A government organisation actively involved in the care and support service is the Woreda HIV/AIDS council, which operates closely with the concerned Woreda administration. With funds from the government and international donors, the council provides beneficiaries with nutrition support, clothing as well as cash for house rent and school fees. It also financially supports bed-ridden AIDS patients. Another major care and support activity the Woreda AIDS council undertakes is home-based care. Through nurses hired at Birr 100 or more, the council sees to it that AIDS patients receive home-based care.

Major grassroots community institutions engaged in HIV/AIDS care and support services are burial association or Iddir. Focus groups of both young PLWHA and community members identified these as key role players in different areas of the campaign. One of these is the care and support service rendered to AIDS patients. In a joint effort with government and NGOs operating in the locality, they distribute food rations and garments to beneficiaries.

The severity of the problem has led to a degree of flexibility and readjustments in community outlook and approach with regard to support for the infected and affected. Pertaining to this, Praag (2000:11) writes: 'The needs of PLWAs are only being partially met by formal health social services, but communities have generated innovative responses to cope with the increased number of patients and to improve the quality of life of PLWAs'. In this connection, an increasing number of burial societies are adopting a policy shift in regards to the timing of due cash payments. Traditionally, the policy of most burial societies was such that, upon the death of a member, a fixed sum of money is paid to his or her family to assist them meet necessities for a period. However, considering the needs and sufferings of AIDS patients over prolonged periods of illness, the practice of paying the money to the family after the death of the patient is being reviewed. A chairperson of a funeral association in the focus group discussion observed that members living and suffering with HIVAIDS have actually not benefited from their affiliation with the institution and the financial contributions that they have made for years towards the strengthening of the institution and mutual support of the entire membership. Instead of the AIDS patients who were committed to burial societies until their death, surviving families have been receiving the financial support, which could have been used to take proper care of deceased members while they were still alive.

Reasons for Failing to Access Existing Care and Support Services

This section attempts to investigate the problems that beneficiaries have experienced in the process of accessing care and support services. Factors that preclude potential users benefiting from available provisions are also considered. Singled out as a principal barrier is the practice of withholding services from persons who are known to be receiving support from a certain provider. Beneficiaries realise the rationale behind the reluctance by providers to serve someone who already has some access to a support system. Care and support agencies often argue that they have difficulties getting enough to distribute. They think they get around the problem by reaching only those not served before and thus limiting the number of beneficiaries. Nevertheless, recipients strongly contend such reasoning by pointing out the circumstances of many support-seekers and the lack of coordination among the support systems. Commenting on this, young male and female PLWHA focus group participants sounded single-minded. They remarked that support services rendered by government and non-government agencies are inadequate, minimal and short-lived. The point on their part is that their HIV/AIDS status is forcing them to become heavily dependent on what they can procure from the care and support networks. Currently, the provisions available at a distribution centres are barely enough for the recipients and those under their care.

Not only are supplies inadequate, but they also lack variety, often being one type of item like wheat, teff, barely, cooking oil, etc. Hence, a beneficiary receiving only one of those items from an agency will not obtain other supplies at a different organisation. But one type of foodstuff is hardly nourishing. The need for rations of higher nutrients is much greater in the case of PLWHA. Especially is this true in view of the value nutritional support has in delaying the onset of full-blown AIDS.

Diversity in the services provided fills the needs of the recipients and promotes the cause of the support programmes. In view of this, beneficiaries suggested better donor coordination and follow up as to the continuity, variety and amount of provisions available. They expressed their preference for a diverse support programme that they indicated has a more practical value. They implied that they need lesser quantities of different items rather than too much of one kind. Thus, they proposed support institutions adopt the approach of one of them focussing on beneficiary needs for a particular form of nutritional supply while another deals with their financial requirements.

A young female participant living with the virus said that doing so has a direct bearing on the effort to control the spread of the virus. Elaborating on this point, she told of an encounter she once had. She began by saying:

One day, I was invited to a wedding party at Crown Hotel. By the time I left the hotel, it was all dark. Luckily, a young man driving a four-wheel vehicle offered me a ride. The driver invited me to sit with him in the front cabin. He greeted me warmly as if we had long known each other. He told me his name and asked if I could tell him mine. Realising his intentions, I introduced myself to him as an active member of Dawn of Hope association of PLWHA. Shocked and stunned, he almost lost control of the car. He remained bereft of speech for some time. When he came back to his senses, he confessed, 'my sister, God bless you! You know I have a wife who is a hostess, and I am a father of four. You spared me great loss and harm'. Dropping me off at my destination, he handed me Birr 50 as an expression of gratitude.

Reports and observations suggest that this experience is not an isolated case. Healthy and attractive looking young PLWHA frequently come into situations where they can lure others or be persuaded to engage in acts of sexual promiscuity. It takes a great deal of social consciousness, humanity and responsible behaviour on their part to resist temptations to engage in sexual practices, especially when the opportunity to make money looks very promising. The young woman quoted earlier suggests that the way to help PLWHA protect themselves and the community in such circumstances is by ensuring that they have access to integrated, consistent, and all-inclusive care and support programmes.

Community representatives who served as key informants for this study observed that NGOs working on HIV/AIDS go about their activities in a less than coordinated fashion. As a result, duplication of programmes exists, a number of agencies concentrating their efforts on certain segments of the population while neglecting others. Strong complaints are voiced in this regard about the coverage given to young people living with the virus in the care and support programmes. According to the key informants, this segment of the community, most affected and threatened as it is by the pandemic, has nevertheless received too little support.

A related problem expressed by these participants is the absence of accurate information about the activities that the various NGOs are undertaking in the fight against the epidemic. The community as well as the beneficiaries are denied the facts concerning service coverage, areas of focus, and type of activities by NGOs involved in the care and support campaign.

Fear of stigma and social isolation is a single major attitudinal factor precluding young PLWHA and AIDS orphans making proper use of existing care and support programmes. In fact, a significant number are inclined or feel freer to access a service when convinced their identity will not be disclosed. For example, most people are encouraged to undergo VCT as an integral part of the general clinical service at health institutions. VCT seekers feel unhindered to visit integrated health centres because onlookers will not directly associate their presence with seeking some type of HIVAIDS oriented assistance. Care and support services are provided largely in the residential areas of the beneficiaries. As a result, many decline to make use of the provisions for fear of being stigmatised by community members as PLWHA.

To qualify for care and support service, PLWHA are required to produce HIV/AIDS certificates and residence identification papers. Failure to meet these requirements has been cited as a chief impediment to accessing existing arrangements. No small number of would-be eligible beneficiaries continues to stay away from support centres as a result. They would rather remain anonymous and miss out on the available services than risk stigmatisation that may accompany processing the required documents.

Trained home-based care agents are greatly involved in the provision of government and non-government sponsored care and support services. These agents are normally fellow community residents of the potential beneficiaries. Rather than risking social discrimination by disclosing their status to the agents and by extension to the community, PLWHA normally prefer to decline to engage with them.

The inadequacy and incompleteness of the provisions have been cited as factors discouraging the young PLWHA from making use of existing arrangements. It was pointed out that the arrangements are not coordinated, one form of care and support excluding other vital components. For example, medical services may not include food provisions without which they mean little, causing beneficiaries not to show interest and motivation in receiving them. Similarly, nutritional support may be provided apart from the payments of house rents, and home-based care without the supply of the necessary furnishings.

Fear of social isolation continues to weigh heavily on the minds of young PLWHA and AIDS patients. Those of them with some possessions or family inheritance strongly favour selling up what they still have and thus survive as long as they can manage, instead of exposing themselves for the sake of receiving care and support.

The inconsistent and sporadic nature of care and support provisions is another reason for the refusal by young PLWHA to join or stay in the programmes. It has been emphasised in the discussions and interviews that especially financial and material forms of support are not provided on a regular basis. They are also hard to predict. Beneficiaries may not be able to anticipate with certainty the next time they are provided. Besides delays, the provisions may be suspended or even terminated without prior notice. Discouraged by the irregularities and uncertainties, beneficiaries may quit, and others who have not yet started will not be motivated.

In too many instances, people become devastated upon realising their status as HIV positive. The state of disappointment and depression causes them to lose purpose and meaning in life for which fundamental reason they generally tend to reject care and support services.

Also obstructing the delivery of HIV/AIDS care and support service are the attitudinal problems reflected by service providers themselves, unwittingly or otherwise. Negative attitudes are reported to prevail at all levels, ranging from the officials and general staff of the concerned government and non-government institutions to professionals specialising in the area. A young male PLWHA reports the following frustrating experience that he had with a Kebele official while applying for cooperation. He said:

> I delivered a supporting letter written on behalf of a fellow PLWHA and myself by Dawn of Hope to the Kebele Administration. The letter requested the administration to consider our circumstance and give us priority so that we could have easy access to a rented home. However, a glance at the subject was enough to irritate him. Looking up, he said to us 'I wish you are not going to ask me for money'. When we told him what we were seeking, he let us move into former latrines now used as dwellings.

Moreover, Kebele administrations are accused of corrupt practices perpetrated against AIDS orphans and vulnerable children. When parents died of HIV/AIDS the orphans have on a number of occasions been made to leave the houses in favour of other occupants. Not only are the orphans denied due support, but what is worse is the abuse committed to promote selfish interests. Members of the administration allegedly negotiate bribes over such houses rather than doing what they can to keep the victims safe and secure.

Many wonder that even places where beneficiaries are supposed to receive the best of care may not after all be the exception to the attitudinal problems reflected by service-providers. The problem manifests itself in different forms. Beneficiaries visiting a health institution for clinical care may be mistreated by whoever is available to provide the service. They could suffer from such things like snubs, scolds or outright insults. Health workers may show themselves fed up of PLWHA, denying them proper care and treatment, as well as demanding more proof for their sero-status than just their official certificates.

Non-governmental organisations engaged in the area of HIV/AIDS may likewise evince wrong attitudes toward the problem as reported by young females living with the virus. They indicated that when they collected monthly allowances at the Organisation for Social Service for AIDS (OSSA), they had to sign with pens apparently meant to be used only by PLWHA. They also alleged that financial support is doled out to them in a manner that betrayed a lack of respect and concern for recipients. Thus, the general mood on the part of the service providers is far from one that makes beneficiaries feel welcome. One of them remarked: 'Their looks seemingly sent the signal that the allowances were handouts after all, and we could take them if we wished, or leave them if we did not'.

Members of all the focus discussion groups have underlined the shortage of medicines as another major problem. They stressed that badly needed medicines are in short supply at government health institutions and available at higher prices at privately owned medical establishments. A great many of them, therefore, fail to obtain medicines that they crucially need due to the shortages at government institutions and their low incomes to buy them elsewhere.

Voluntary Counselling and Testing (VCT) service is another problem area reported. Not all those who may present themselves for the service may necessarily get it. In addition, once they are diagnosed as HIV positive, a counselling service they were promised to encourage them for a test may prove to be not as satisfying as expected. It is not also unusual to be served by VCT councillors whose competence is questioned by beneficiaries. Also mentioned was the quality of facilities at VCT centres. There are allegations that some receive incorrect test results, contributing to fewer people accessing the service.

Restrictions on the category of users are also regarded as a problem in accessing VCT service. In certain neighbourhoods it is said that only commercial sex workers are eligible for VCT. This excludes other community groups in the area from the service. The effort to keep the public informed on the necessity and availability of VCT service has allegedly been insufficient. Despite it being an integral part of the continuum of the HIV/AIDS care and support system, the views and remarks of many suggest that it has nevertheless not been given its due attention. Other problems reported are insufficient number of testing centres at reasonable distances, inadequate public awareness about the necessity and benefit of VCT, limited post-test social and psychological support, shortage of the necessary cash to undergo tests, and irregularities and lack of consistency in the delivery of pre- and post-test counselling services.

Observations are also made of constraints related to the delivery of home-based care. First, home-based agents may not be readily available when needed largely because they are volunteers, doing other jobs to earn a living. Besides the shortage of time and inconvenience as a result, voluntary HBC agents may move to other places for occupational reasons and therefore suspend service provision. Others may interrupt their voluntary work compelled by lack of both consistent training and materials needed for service delivery. Some quit because they are disturbed and discouraged by the deteriorating health condition of patients in their care. Lack of acceptance by beneficiaries has also been cited as a reason why certain home-based agents have discontinued or withdrawn from the service. It is reported that PLWHA tend to reject HBC agents familiar to them or living in the same residential neighbourhoods for fear they will disclose their identity to community members, causing them to become stigmatised and socially isolated.

To sum up, it seems appropriate to quote some comments on the issue by Praag (2000:11):

> Care and empathy for PLWAs are lacking or inaccessible in many parts of the world. Even when health facilities are available, operational and attitudinal problems limit utilization and access to quality care. For example, in East Africa dispensaries and health centres are the first level clinical contact facilities available. These levels are virtually bypassed by people with HIV-related illness for various reasons, including lack of drugs, fear of disclosure of sero-status within the community and poor diagnostic knowledge of HIV-related illness among staff.

Self-Help as a Coping Strategy

PLWHA have developed a number of mechanisms to help them cope with the virus and the stigma associated with it. These mechanisms include tactical or strategic disclosure (disclosing status where care and support may be available and declining to do so where stigma is anticipated) and joining PLWHA networks.

Most PLWHA tend to combine these two strategies to deal with the socioeconomic and psychological consequences of HIV/AIDS. A great number of those involved in the study depended on support provided by relatives, care and support organisations, and associations of PLWHA.

More than half of the PLWHA who participated in the study disclosed their sero-status to someone they trusted, close relatives in great many cases. The outcome has largely been such that they received emotional and practical support after revealing their circumstances. The following statements illustrate that as a direct result of the expressions of sympathy and other kinds of support these PLWHA have succeeded in their efforts to cope with the virus effectively.

When my husband discovered I was HIV positive, he was far from tolerant. He chased me out of home and I had no one to turn to except my brother. Contrary to my expectations, my brother responded favourably when I shared my secrets with him. The concern and sympathies he showed me helped me greatly to overcome my feelings of loneliness and increased my confidence that I have someone on my side who I can rely on in moments of deep emotional turmoil (A young married female PLWHA).

It has now been four years since I learned of my status as HIV positive. For the first two years of this period, I kept the secret to myself suffering the consequences alone. After two years though I revealed my status to my mother and sister who, against all anticipations, came to my rescue and took a deep interest in my personal well-being. They responded positively and immediately, extending all emotional and other forms of care and support to the extent they could. This has been the main factor that prolonged my life for the following four years. Without their care and support, I would likely have died much earlier (A young male PLWHA).

Joining care and support organisations and associations of PLWHA as a means of self-help is another of the coping mechanisms used. These networks have proved to be a source of emotional, material and financial support for the PLWHA. They have also been channels of communication whereby information, care and counselling continue to be available to beneficiaries. The practical value particularly of membership in the associations lies in the fact that the PLWHA find a conducive environment that facilitates the sharing of common concerns and sentiments without hindrance. The favourable conditions created by the associations benefit the members by giving them hope for the future and sense of purpose in living that promote an optimistic outlook on life.

An additional practical advantage of membership in the associations of PLWHA and accessing provisions from care and support organisations is that they create forums whereby those living with the virus come together and know each other closely. Prior to joining these bodies, most PLWHA rarely knew another person who lived with the virus. That created the feeling in most of them that they were the only ones who had contracted the virus. The interviews conducted indicate that not knowing another individual sharing the same problem led PLWHA to the mistaken belief that they are a unique people because of the virus and have little hope for success and enjoyment. However, the opportunities that the networks offered them to come together and share experiences helped to correct their wrong views and perceptions of themselves, enabling them to cope with their circumstances in a more realistic and practical fashion.

On this note, responses from focus group discussions and individual interviews overwhelmingly indicate that people whom PLWHA consider especially understanding and sympathetic towards them are fellow HIV positive individuals. The following cases illustrate the valuable role played by networks in the lives of the PLWHA:

> After testing positive for HIV, I could not control my tears and emotions. I was crying loudly, not caring about whoever was there around me. I was more concerned with my children than with myself, believing that there was no one who would support and provide for them. But a young woman who happened to be at the clinic came over and consoled me. She identified herself with me telling me that she too was HIV positive. Assuring me that there were also many other people who live with the virus as I did, she promised to put me in contact with them and facilitate my membership in one of their associations. Her words of consolation helped me pull my thoughts together and stay calm. At the association, I met a number of HIV positive persons with whom I easily mingled and shared personal experiences. I realised that I was not the only one living with the virus. Besides information, the association has enabled me access emotional, medical and other practical support (A young female living with the virus).

> I keep talking about the virus with high degree of openness with my friends who are also infected. The more we talk about it, our knowledge about the virus increases and to that extent we learn how to cope with its consequences (A young female PLWHA).

> At first, I was reluctant to go to the association of PLWHA, despite the constant advice of my counsellor. I talked to my brother about what I was facing, who then brought me in contact with Mekdim Ethiopia Association of PLWHA. There, I made many friends who also live with the virus as I do myself. Gradually, we became very close to each other, discussing our situation frankly. Especially am I an intimate friend of three members of the association who enjoy an unusual type of company and friendship. We are quick to support each other when one of us is ill or gets into some kind of trouble. Enjoying such special relationships has helped us build cooperative sprit and mutual trust and confidence. It has also shaped our attitudes toward the reality, making it possible for us to accept our circumstance and live with it comfortably rather than trying to dismiss it as if it were not true (A young, divorced woman).

However, even more important than the practical support, as the PLWHA say, is the emotional help that they access through professional counselling, training, as well as the constructive interaction among themselves. A female PLWHA who joined Mekdim Ethiopia after living with the virus in seclusion for five years describes as follows the positive change she has experienced:

I came to know of my sero-status as far back as 2000. But I could not make up my mind on the question of joining a PLWHA association or applying to care and support institutions. I chose to rely on the practical and emotional help that my family provided. That kept me going safe and sound for as long as three years. During this entire period, I knew no other person who lived with the virus and so I thought of myself as one of the exceptional people who contracted it. Although my relatives were considerate and supportive toward me, we never brought up the issue of my being HIV positive for open and direct discussion. Meanwhile, a turn of events came in my situation in the middle of 2003 when I was suddenly taken ill. My health deteriorated so badly that I thought my final moments of life had at last arrived. The emotional and physical sufferings that resulted from the critical stages of my illness were so excruciating that I nearly decided to commit suicide to avoid further agony. Seeing my condition was terrible and that it needed emotional support besides medical care, a physician advised my relatives to take me to one of the associations of PLWHA. Once I became a member Mekdim Ethiopia, my overall condition improved progressively. For one thing, there I met many people who lived with the virus like myself and shared common interests, experiences and feelings with me (A young girl PLWHA).

PLWHA said that professional counselling was one important aspect of the services provided by the associations and the care and support institutions that brought real benefits in the process of coping with their circumstances. They added that those PLWHA who received intensive counselling and others with adequate training in counselling and home-based care performed a great deal better in coping behaviour than those without this exposure.

Needs and Problems of AIDS Orphans

As stated earlier, children numbering in the tens of thousands have already been orphaned as a result of AIDS in Addis Ababa. It has been forecast that huge numbers will still be orphaned over the coming decade as people continue to die from AIDS-related causes in their child-rearing ages. Thus, orphan-hood being an important facet of the overall national crisis caused by the pandemic, no prevention and control effort is ever complete without duly addressing this growing social menace.

Focus group discussions were conducted in order to identify the problems that AIDS orphans experience under different circumstances. Involved in the discussions were community members as well as AIDS orphans themselves benefiting from some kind of care and support programmes.

The children of people living with HIV/AIDS (PLWHA) and AIDS patients are probably the ones who bear the largest brunt of the HIV/AIDS scourge next to their parents. The impact of the pandemic is known to be multi-faceted, exposing such children to a multiplicity of problems which continue to become more intense and diversified following the loss of either parent or both to the disease. Whether the children are aware of it or not, the prospect of orphan-hood is imminent, especially once the HIV/AIDS positive parents begin to manifest the symptoms of full-blown AIDS. Upon parental loss, the orphans are most likely to be stigmatised in connection with the deaths believed or widely suspected to have resulted from AIDS. It is not uncommon to assume that AIDS orphans themselves carry the virus just because they lost their parents to it. The orphans, therefore, risk becoming the objects of stigma and discrimination by community members, neighbours, peers, and, in no few cases, even close relatives.

Whatever assistance and cooperation the parents used to receive from relatives and associates is very likely to cease after their death, leaving surviving children without care and support. Further compounding the difficulties of the orphans is the failure of the parents to make the necessary arrangements that help the children to cope with the circumstances of orphan-hood. Practice has revealed that parents in a great many cases do not seem to pay much attention to the fate of their children after their death. The problems that AIDS orphans experience in connection with the right to inheritance of family property, land or otherwise, give a clear and strong indication of this fact. Thus, not only do AIDS orphans have difficulties finding relatives coming to their rescue, but to make matters worse, they risk losing part or all of their property rights to those putting forward illegitimate claims.

In desperation, a great number of orphans land up on the streets in an attempt to find food by doing menial jobs or begging. Girls become obliged to sell their labour as domestic servants and exchange sexual favours for cash. While orphaned boys and girls may somehow keep themselves going in this way, street life only increases their vulnerability to a range of further and more complex troubles. The street milieu exposes the orphans to high sexual activity, wilful or forced, with great likelihood of contracting the HIV virus, besides sliding into a number of harmful practices. Children in such situations are hardly able to continue schooling, putting their prospects for a normal life at even higher risk.

While many of the problems cited are common to orphaned boys and girls there are also some that are markedly gender-specific. Upon the death of parents, the responsibilities for the care of the household falls primarily on girls, who thus become burdened with carrying out the bulk of domestic activities. Besides being physically demanding, assuming a leading role in domestic life also takes a heavy toll on the psychology and emotions of the girls in charge. The pressures often become unbearably intense, compelling the girls to seek a way out by practising commercial sex. However, they can feed themselves and their siblings in this way neither adequately nor perpetually. Sex work not only deprives them of their self-respect and sense of decency, but also heightens their exposure to unwanted pregnancies and the chance of infection with STDs including HIV/AIDS. Moreover, acts of sexual violence including rape perpetrated against these girls while still at home or once out in the streets are very likely.

AIDS Orphan Care and Support Services

Currently, a limited number of faith-based and non-government institutions are reported to be active in Addis Ababa in the area of care and support services for AIDS orphans. This study investigated the activities that these institutions and the two associations of PLWHA in the country are carrying out. These are the 'Counselling and Social Services Centre of the Medical Missionary of Mary (MMM)', 'St. Mary's Orphan Support Programme' of the Daughters of Charity of the Ethiopian Catholic Church, 'Yehiwot Tesfa Counselling and Social Services Centre' of the Ethiopian Evangelical Church of Mekane Yesus, as well as Dawn of Hope and Mekdim Ethiopia associations of PLWHA.

Information was gathered on the types of services provided through interviews with the staff of the institutions and focus group discussions with beneficiary orphans. This component of the research revealed that the existing care and support services targeting AIDS orphans basically include food, shelter, and clothing provisions, health care, psychological support and supplies of educational and related material. The institutions provide food rations to the orphans whose living circumstances vary according to their particular experiences. There are those who remain in an extended family setting despite the loss of one parent or both to HIV/AIDS. Others find themselves in child-headed households, in which case the eldest of the surviving children usually takes over responsibilities following the death of the parents. The institutions also make arrangements for orphaned children to share group homes in situations where there are no close relatives to take them into their homes, or the orphans have for different reasons lost shelter as well. The food rations include wheat, famiex, and cooking oil. It is reported that the food rations given to the beneficiaries in extended family structure do not get them through to the next round of monthly rationing. The insufficiency is attributed to the limited amounts of food aid made available to the institutions by donor agencies. However, the centres report that they make every possible effort to see to it that orphans in group homes obtain regular and sufficient food provisions at reasonable time intervals. The Yehiwot Tesfa, one of such institutions, provides cash rather than food items with which the beneficiaries or their guardians themselves buy food supplies.

Clothing and school uniforms are provided to the orphans once a year. They are also given money to pay house rent, and in the case of those in group homes, the institutions settle the house rents.

The orphans are also provided with basic health services mostly at clinics operated by the care and support institutions. The poor living conditions of the children generally make them vulnerable to different parasitic and infectious diseases such as typhoid and diarrhoea. The nurses at the clinics treat the children for these and other illnesses, referring major cases to higher health institution for further medication. The centres cover the medical costs of the referral cases.

Psychological support makes up a significant component in the care and support programmes that the institutions are implementing. This type of service is vitally important to children who have experienced the loss of parents in their tender years. The grief and distress associated with the bereavement results in emotional disturbance and stress that the surviving children find beyond their means to cope with. Their depression is further aggravated by the difficulties they continue to experience in their efforts to get on with life and adjust to their losses. A single dominant expression of their psychological state is the behavioural problems that they tend to exhibit around the home and beyond. The institutions identify orphans with special care and support needs in this area by way of information gathered from family members and close neighbours. Once identified, they are given counselling services through regular home visits or by appointments at the counselling centres.

As well as the aforementioned services, orphans in these programmes also receive educational support to ensure that they continue schooling despite their circumstances. The educational support involves supplies of school materials and uniforms and the payment of school fees. Yehiwot Tesfa provides the cash to enable beneficiaries get the needed supplies, handing out Birr 50 monthly per child for educational materials, and Birr 200 annually for school uniforms and shoes. A school fee of another Birr 120 is also allocated for each beneficiary.

Through negotiations with the concerned school administrations, arrangements are made by the institutions so that school fees are waived for orphan children. For motivational purposes, students with the best performances are awarded prizes in the form of cash or educational materials. In addition, the institutions support the orphans in connection with their rights to property inheritance. This is reported to be one of the major problems that AIDS orphans encounter and need external assistance to properly handle. Therefore, the organisations discussed in this study incorporate into their programmes some support for beneficiaries with regard to property rights. First, they approach responsible members of the extended family to address smoothly the dispute. If that fails, an effort is made to peacefully resolve it by involving in the matter a committee of elders close or acceptable to the family. In extreme cases, the institutions take the case to organisations who can lend legal support so that the property rights of the orphans are respected in courts of law.

The majority of the orphans receiving care and support services in these institutions are known to live with members of the extended families. This is in line with the policies of the government and organisations catering to the needs of AIDS orphans. These bodies encourage community-based care and support rather than institutionalised support systems such as orphanages, which should only be a last resort.

Thus, the centres take the necessary measures to contact the closest relatives of their clients who have died of HIV/AIDS and leaving children behind. The purpose is to persuade the relatives to take over the responsibility for the care of the orphans. There are times when family members of the deceased may of their own initiative approach the institutions in the hope that the support will continue after the death of the client and that they can now access it by fostering the surviving child. In other circumstances, the children of the deceased clients themselves may connect family members with the care and support institutions.

However, whatever the means of contact, family members respond differently with regard to care of the orphans. Some have gone as far as offering to take the child away into rural villages where they themselves reside. Moving to live and grow up in a strange environment can, however, have undesirable effects on the child, as experience has shown. The maladjustment, coupled with the psychological stress resulting from the parental loss, could make things extremely difficult, seriously affecting the future prospects of the orphan in care. Nevertheless, a most widely observed response by family members is unwillingness to commit themselves to the care of the orphans and accept them as part of their family. In fact, there are some who deny any blood relationships or simply disappear after realising the cause of the death and the intentions of the institution.

When no family member is thus committed, the centres make alternative arrangements to ensure the orphans get the necessary care and support. They arrange for the orphans to live in groups in rented houses where a foster mother is employed for them to take care of their day-to-day needs. Group homes enable orphans to learn to manage their lives independently, gain experience through social interaction, and grow up in the community where they were born, without socially dislocated and therefore needing assistance with the process of readjustment.

Other than group homes, arrangements are made for adoption to take care of orphans who are not in a position to live with their extended families. Accordingly, the institutions receive and process requests from interested adopters or themselves initiate contacts in a bid to find potential adoptive families. They make adoption arrangements for the children both with families within the country or abroad. Before an adoption takes place, however, certain issues need to be addressed. First, the personal choice of the potential adopters in regards to the age and sex of the adoptees has to be considered as a matter of priority. The government is also involved in the process through the Child and Youth Affairs Department of the Ministry of Labour and Social Affairs and the grassroots unit of city government, the Kebele Administration. The former issues approval for the adoption to take place after considering the case from the legal and administrative points of view. Based on the information from witnesses, the Kebele Administration must confirm in a supporting letter that a child is genuinely an AIDS orphan for the process of adoption to commence. It is the role of the care and support centres to follow up on the progress by maintaining regular contacts with potential adopters, foreign or domestic, via correspondence and other means.

As already suggested, institutional care for orphans should only be arranged as a final option, having exhausted all possibilities to arrange for them to live with extended or adoptive families. However, institutional care becomes a necessity in situations where none of the aforementioned arrangements proves to be practical. Thus, a resort to orphanage becomes inevitable in the absence of extended family members showing an interest in taking care of the orphans, or when there are disparities between potential adoptive parents and children needing care, or with the physical and emotional inability of the orphans to stay in a group home setting. Compelled by these circumstances, the Counselling Centre of the Medical Missionary of Mary (MMM) alone reports having placed up to thirty children in an orphanage.

Orphan care and support furnishes an important form of service rendered by the associations of PLWHA, Dawn of Hope and Mekdim Ethiopia. To provide a service, the associations first investigate whether an orphan lost one parent or both due to AIDS. Once they establish AIDS as a cause of orphan-hood, they enrol the victims as association members. Following this, an assessment will be carried out about felt needs of the orphans through group counselling and discussion. Accordingly, the following services will be available to eligible orphan beneficiaries:

(i) For orphans living with the virus there is nutritional support and provision of house rent and medical care.

(ii) For orphans needing in-house care, nurses are hired to cook their food and do their cleaning. Dawn of Hope is at the moment caring for twenty AIDS orphans through hired nurses and guardians at a group home organised for this purpose.

(iii) For school age orphans a supply of educational materials and school uniforms are provided twice a year.

(iv) For orphans tested HIV negative, arrangements for adoption with interested volunteers, local or foreign, may be made. In this effort, Dawn of Hope has made adoption arrangements for a number of such orphans in the United States.

(v) On public holidays arrangements are made marking major holidays such as Christmas, Eastern, New Year's Day, Id Al Fater (Ramadan) so that orphans may celebrate them as the rest of the community do. With funds raised from different sources, special foods are served besides some cash provision to assist the beneficiaries.

Summary and Recommendations

Summary

On the basis of the information obtained from young people living with HIV/ AIDS and AIDS orphans, their most important needs can be stated to be health care — physical, socioeconomic, and psychological. Thus, they singled out as the first high priority need for the provision of affordable, comprehensive and specialised medical service. The study population emphasised the importance of tailoring the proposed health services to the needs and conditions of the targeted beneficiaries. This suggests that the packages be inclusive of the treatment of opportunistic infections, counselling and psychological support, and home-based care and nursing.

The study participants prioritised physical and socio-economic needs as the second most important. Low standards of living, poverty, and the weakening of the body's immune system are reported to aggravate these needs. Provisions of a physical and socioeconomic nature basically encompass nutritional support, and supplies of shelter and clothing. The nutritional aspect of such support stands out as the most prominent since it plays an important role in strengthening the body's resistance to infection and improving the health condition of the infected. The need for decent housing has been described as the next biggest. Evictions from rented houses and hardship in maintaining or securing a new one are among common stories forming the pattern of mistreatment that young PLWHA often experience at the hands of house owners and neighbours. Particularly is this the case with AIDS orphans. Quite often, they are left homeless upon the death of their parents. Reportedly, those who rent out houses — public and private alike — resort to forcing helpless orphan children out of their shelters once their parents have passed away. To make matters worse, their plight may not end there. Dislocated from their once secure abode, the victims often find themselves vulnerable to various forms of abuse, including sexual assaults in the case of orphan girls. Homelessness also generally causes these orphans to go out to the streets, where they are exposed to a number of risks, contracting HIV/AIDS being a most likely one.

Emotional and psychological needs come fourth in order of priorities that young PLWHA and AIDS orphans underscored in the course of the study. It was not difficult to gauge from a reading of their responses the extent of their hunger for social acceptance and expressions of empathy. They expressed a general feeling that the rehabilitation component of the national HIV/AIDS policy has not gone far enough in addressing such critical needs. This is shown by the fact that the available care and support services dealing with this aspect of the problem prove to be inadequate compared with the size of the existing demand.

The other point of focus in this study has to do with the existing care and support services for young PLWHA and AIDS orphans in Addis Ababa. Thus, a survey was made of such institutions operational at the time of the study. According to the information provided by the beneficiaries, the associations of PLWHA, Dawn of Hope and Mekdim Ethiopia carry out the largest percentage of care and support activities in the metropolis. The major aspect of the service rendered is constituted by professional HIV/AIDS counselling and psychological support. Other types of services the associations provide include material support, orphan care, legal support, home-based care, and financial assistance to cover medical costs. Home-based care (HBC) in particular continues to be one of the chief areas of focus to which these associations are attaching ever-greater importance. Both the caregivers and recipients stand to benefit from the great emphasis laid on HBC, as they themselves acknowledged. The job opportunities created as a result of this type of service enable members of the associations to gain access to gainful employment. Moreover, the caregivers, who are themselves HIV-positive, will be in a position to serve others under like circumstances with such empathy and commitment that the nature of the job demands.

Community members who participated in this study identified government and non-government agencies, Community-Based Organisations (CBOs), youth associations and anti-AIDS clubs as the other bodies that play an important role in the provision of care and support services to PLWHA and AIDS orphans.

Voluntary Counselling and Testing (VCT) is reported to constitute an important part of the continuum of care and support services provided by indigenous and international NGOs. Key informants and focus group discussion participants singled out the NGOs that are actively involved in this type of service. These are Mary Joy through Development, Medical Missionary of Mary Counselling and Social Service Centre (MMM), Hiwot Tesfa, Organisation for Social Service for AIDS (OSSA), and CARE Ethiopia. The information obtained shows that VCT services are available to AIDS orphans and vulnerable children for free, and only at token payments to other clients.

The city government is also involved in the provision of care and support services to young PLWHA and AIDS orphans. The HIV/AIDS Council, which body is structured at sub-city level, utilises resources made available by the government and donor agencies to meet the needs especially of those with full-blown AIDS. Besides nutritional support, the council makes cash provision to cover housing, clothing and medical expenses. It also ensures the deployment of nurses to carry out HBC activities. In addition, the AIDS Council operates, in collaboration with the Kebele administration, Iddir societies and youth associations, to conduct Information, Education, and Communication (IEC) programmes.

Grass-root organisations, Iddir (burial societies) in particular, are gaining increased prominence in relation to their involvement in HIV/AIDS-based care and support programmes. As well as playing an active role in community sensitisation and educational campaigns against the pandemic, burial societies contribute a good measure of socioeconomic and material support to the infected and orphaned. Burial societies have also become an important force in another way in the effort to halt the spread of HIV infection. Agencies involved in the delivery of care and support services use the leverage that these grassroots institutions command over community members to promote their programmes.

This study has also dealt with problems that PLWHA and AIDS orphans encounter as they try to access existing care and support services. Clients observed that inadequacy and duplication of services and lack of coordination among providers are some of the constraints they experience. The shortage of clear information and non-transparency concerning which agency is providing what type of service is another problem cited. Failure to access such information is said to have hindered effective utilisation of the existing continuum of care and support services. Moreover, beneficiaries brought up the point that their actual felt needs are not usually taken into consideration in the designing and implementation of programmes meant to address their problems.

The study population expressed in strong terms their dissatisfaction regarding the scarcity of drugs for the treatment of opportunistic infections. Even when available, anti-retrovirals continue to be unaffordable for most of those in need of them. They also stressed as a major shortcoming the state of low public awareness about the need for voluntary counselling and testing, and the continuing general reluctance to access the existing VCT service.

Recommendations

Young PLWHA, AIDS orphans and community members who participated in this study have made the following recommendations regarding the necessary remedial measures to adopt in order to improve the quality and size of the current care and support programmes.

(i) Facilitating the necessary conditions for the provision of comprehensive medical care to young PLWHA, AIDS orphans and affected families. Supply of antiretrovirals at subsidised prices.

(ii) Making available sufficient nutritional support.

(iii) Ensuring that they find decent homes or supporting them financially to pay house rents.

(iv) Making provision of materials, clothing, and home furnishings as the need may be.

(v) Training family members in the delivery of care and support.

(vi) Making the necessary arrangements for the provision of regular and consistent counselling services. Offering counselling service at individual home level. Establishing social committees to deal with the psychological problems of young PLWHA and AIDS orphans.

(vii) Enabling PLWHA take care of themselves through the provision of skill training to those capable of active engagements and their family members.

(viii) Encouraging community participation at all levels in this endeavour from planning to evaluation.

(ix) Ensuring that the effort is coordinated in collaboration with government and NGOs and CBOs in the area.

(x) Strengthening the home-based care service by way of sufficient training and material incentive to the agents. Building their capacities through refresher courses and updates on current information about HIV/AIDS.

(xi) Support to orphans and vulnerable children so that they will not quit or drop out of school. Skill training to those old enough to take up a job. Additional educational support outside school.

References

Teklu, A., 1991, 'Knowledge, Attitudes, and Practice Study on Sexual Practices Related to HIV Transmission and Prevention among Male Residents of Arba Minch Town', Southwest Ethiopia, M.PH. Thesis, Department of Community Health, Faculty of Medicine, University of Addis Ababa.

Abrhaley, T., 2001, 'School Youth Awareness Creation on HIV/AIDS by Indigenous NGOs: The Case of National Aid and Rehabilitation Centre (NARC)', Senior Essay in Sociology, Addis Ababa University.

Addis Ababa City Administration Health Bureau (AACAHB), 1999, 'HIV/AIDS in Addis Ababa: Background, Projections, Impacts and Intervention', Addis Ababa.

Addisu, S., 2001, 'The Socioeconomic Impact of HIV/AIDS on Iddirs with Particular Reference to Iddirs in Woreda 11', *Senior Essay in Sociology*, Addis Ababa University.

Alem E., 2002, 'Problems of AIDS-orphaned Female Students in Some Selected Elementary and Secondary Schools in Addis Ababa', Senior Essay, Department of Educational Planning and Management, Faculty of Education, Addis Ababa University.

Alemu A., 2002, 'A Study on the Attitude, Knowledge, Belief and Practice of Students of Higher Learning Institutions Towards HIV/AIDS: The Case of Kotebe College of Teacher Education (KCTE)', Senior Essay in Sociology, Addis Ababa University.

Alemu A., 2000, The Awareness of Adolescents Towards HIV/AIDS: Its Spread and Consequences (A Case Study of Menelik II Secondary School)' BA Thesis. Department of Geography, Addis Ababa University.

Anannia A., 2000, Coping with AIDS: The Social Dimension of the Epidemic in Selected Areas of Addis Ababa, MA Thesis in Social Anthropology, Addis Ababa University.

Anannia A., 2002, 'Coping with the Challenges of AIDS: The Experience of Persons Living with HIV/AIDs in Addis Ababa', Northeast African Studies (forthcoming).

Ayalew G., 2002, 'Community Perceptions, Attitudes and Treatment of Sexually Transmitted Diseases (STDs) in Bahr Dar Town', Northeast African Studies (forthcoming).

Central Statistical Authority, 1999, 'Report on the 1998 Health and Nutrition Survey', Addis Ababa.

Converse, P, Wuhib, T., Mulatu, M. S. et al., 2002, 'Bibliography of HIV/AIDS in Ethiopia and Ethiopians in the Diaspora', Ethiopian Journal of Health Development, in press.

Kloos, H. and Damen H.M., 2002, 'Selected Community Organizations and Agents and Poverty Reduction Programs in HIV/AIDS Prevention and Control in Ethiopia', Northeast African Studies (forthcoming).

National AIDS Council (NAC), 2001, Strategic Framework for National Response to HIV/AIDS. Addis Ababa.

Nebiyu, G., 2001, 'The Socioeconomic and Psychological Impacts of HIV/AIDS on the People Living with the Virus: with Particular Reference to Dawn of Hope Association', Senior Essay in Sociology, Addis Ababa University.

Ministry of Health, 2000, AIDS in Ethiopia, Addis Ababa: Ethiopian Ministry of Health.

UNAIDS, 2000, 'The Epidemiology of HIV/AIDS in Ethiopia: A Review', Addis Ababa: UNAIDS/WHO.

UNAIDS, 2002, Report on the Global HIV/AIDS Epidemic, Geneva: UNAIDS.

Zinabu A., 1999, 'Knowledge, Attitude and Behaviour (KAB) on HIV/AIDS/ STDs Among Workers in the Informal Sector in Addis Ababa', MSc. Thesis, Demographic Training and Research Centre, Addis Ababa University.

Sexuality and HIV/AIDS Among Young Residents of Mafalala Barrio, Maputo, Mozambique

Margarida Paulo

Introduction

This paper aims to understand the issue of sexuality among the young residents of Mafalala Barrio, Maputo, in Mozambique, and contribute to HIV/AIDS educational programmes in this locality and elsewhere.

HIV/AIDS educational programmes argue that providing the youth with correct information about HIV/AIDS infection and prevention will help them to make responsible and sensitive decisions about their health, which will reduce the spread of HIV/AIDS in the country (Inquérito Nacional de Estatísticas, INE 2001, 2002; Geração Biz 2001 and Population Services International, PSI, 2001, 1999, 1998). The INE points out that 37,736 young people were HIV/AIDS positive in 1998-1999, a figure which increased to 65,144 HIV/AIDS infections in 2000-2002. Clearly, these data should make us rethink and question the efficacy of the methods used so far in HIV/AIDS educational programmes.

In trying to understand the perception of sexuality among young people and the reasons why they do not accept the message that they should practise 'safe sex', I focus on various socio-cultural factors. These relate to families in Mozambique following the country's independence in 1975 and the end of the civil war in 1994, which resulted in the peace agreement between Frelimo and Renamo in Rome.

The foregoing provides a brief introduction to this study. The next section will present the methodology and ethical considerations.

Methodology and Ethical Considerations

The fieldwork was conducted in two stages. The first stage took place from 12 to 22 November 2003. As a young black woman, fluent in Portuese, the language used among my informants, it was possible for me to enter into the everyday lives of the young women in Mafalala barrio. My research assistant, José Bambo,[1] on the other hand, gathered information on the young men's experiences, because it would have been easier for him as a man to interact with them. The second stage of the fieldwork took place between 5 January and 22 February, 2004. During these two stages, I collected twenty-seven life histories, with particular emphasis on issues of dating and sexuality, of which I only analysed ten in-depth.

Initially, while preparing for the fieldwork I was not clear what age group I should work with. I thus followed Wyn and White (1995:11), who explained that 'youth is a relational concept because it exists and has meaning largely in relation to the concept of adulthood'. This argument suggests that there is no definition of 'youth' that would suit all contexts. Within the context of my own data, 'young' refers to people aged between 20 and 24 years old. Their educational level varied from grade five to grade ten. The informants who participated in my fieldwork were primarily students, domestic workers, businessmen and women in the Adelina market[2] and in other parts of Maputo City, although two of the young men did not reveal their activities.

I mainly used qualitative methods such as life histories, as discussed by De Queiroz et al., (1988), Tierney (2000) and Thomas and Znaniecki (1958) in conjunction with participant observation, as used by Bernard (1995), as participant observation may be ineffective on its own, as demonstrated by Angrosimo and Pérez (2000). In addition, I visited Machaca,[3] a youth organisation created in 1996 to respond to the HIV/AIDS epidemic in the barrio. During the interviews I did not use a tape recorder because it was not convenient to record young people's experiences when they were washing clothes, playing timbila,[4] going to the market and walking around. Although the tape recorder is theoretically one of the best ways of recording interviews, its use requires special attention to ethical issues. Informants must be educated about the use and purpose of the tape recorder, and the recording itself must be openly made, which can be distracting. Instead, my research assistant José Bambo and I recorded the interviews by thorough note-taking.

Taking the life histories of young people proved to be a particularly useful method, because they spontaneously raised issues that concerned them. It also created opportunities for in-depth research, and allowed a relationship of trust to develop between researcher and informants. In this way, the following research questions were addressed by this study:

- What is sexuality?
- How do young people view HIV/AIDS prevention campaigns?

Participant observation, too, was useful because it allowed me to compare the information presented by young people during the interview with actual practices among family and friends. Participant observation was also helpful because it made it possible to observe the youth during the day and at night, to see what they do and say, and what they do not do or say.

There are strong debates around ethical issues in social science, particularly as concerns the conduct of research (see Caplan 2003; Nyamnjoh 2007). Although there is little consensus among anthropologists in different contexts, anthropological ethics does highlight the relevance of protecting informants. I thus retained the anonymity of my informants, as suggested by the American Anthropological Association's statements on ethical issues (1971).[5] I was aware that the results of the research might border on the pornographic due to the nature of the topic and that I might also create negative impressions of the young residents of Mafalala barrio. This study does not however intend to increase discrimination against young residents of Mafalala. Rather, it attempts to improve our understanding of the perceptions of sexuality among young people in order to understand how HIV/AIDS educational programmes could achieve better results in Mozambique.

This section has described the methodology and ethical considerations. The next section will provide the context of post-civil war Mozambique, the consequent fragmentation of family structure, and the implications for HIV campaigns.

The Context of Post-civil War Mozambique, the Consequent Fragmentation of Family Structure, and Implications for HIV Campaigns

In the social sciences, the concept of 'family' has at times created controversy. It has resisted attempts to universalise or to describe any kind of normative family, in any culture. For example, in industrial societies the definition of 'family' has meant a man, a woman, and their children — a 'nuclear' family. This view tends to be exclusive: other persons are not seen as part of the family structure even if they share the same space. Over time, the concept of family had to expand to embrace more complex arrangements, not to mention diverse ideals about what it means to belong to a family.

By contrast, in non-industrialised societies, 'family' tends to be accepted as more inclusive, an 'extended' family. In this type of family, a couple, their children, cousins, nephews and in-laws are part of the same family structure. It is clear that there is no single definition of 'family' that can characterise it in all contexts.

In Mozambique, the concept of family becomes contradictory, most particularly in urban areas. Although some families are nuclear, economically advantaged families continue to sustain their extended family in the urban context, and clearly view the economically disadvantaged members as family. The ruling Frelimo (Mozambique Liberation Front) party added further contradictions when after the independence of Mozambique from colonial power Portugal in 1975, the government adopted a Marxist-Leninist policy towards family life (Paulo 2003, 1998; Arnfred, 2001). Based on this political philosophy, the government forbade some key local practices that had sustained African families: notably the practice of lobolo or bride price and ritual initiation. The goal, it appeared, was to create 'a new man' who was free of capitalist values (including local family values) and did not engage in exploitative relationships, including within the family.

Although the government had forbidden these practices, families continued to pay lobolo and initiate youth. As a result, in 1987 the government came up with new policies that were more realistic and tolerant of local traditions. During this period, the media played a role in showing the shift in the political arena, by giving space to ceremonies such as guaza muthini, a traditional ceremony performed close to a river in Marracuene district, Maputo. This ceremony is carried out every year in order to ensure land fertility. The return to local practices is also experienced in the inauguration of roads and companies. Seeing these local ceremonies conducted in the public context with government approval, people realised that they too could be free to perform their own ceremonies without any fear.

It may be that the concept of family, however it is defined, is too limiting to be useful, except in terms of political economy. The anthropological term 'kinship' is more promising as a linguistic tool to assist the discussion on sexuality and HIV/AIDS prevention campaigns in Mozambique.

The 'kinship' approach provides an understanding of the diversity of social practices, and of the meanings people give and expect from each other within groups (see Fortes 1969; Fox 1967; Gillespie 2000; Goody 1969, 1973). This being the case, it is useful to describe two types of kinship system in Mozambique. The matrilineal kinship system characterises families in Northern Mozambique, and the patrilineal kinship system is a key feature of families in Southern Mozambique.

In these kinship systems people reacted differently to changes in the political economy of the country, and the ideological assault on their values and practices. The kinship system to which they belong also strongly influences people in the ways they think about relationships, protection and sexuality. However, the kinship influence on people's everyday life does vary according to gender, age, religion and location within social networks.

I will start with the description of the matrilineal kinship system. In this system, couples are expected to marry and then stay on the woman's family land. The man is supposed to work on his in-laws' land, and has no claim to any land rights or ownership until he has children, particularly girls. Daughters are valued in this system, because if they are successfully married, they might bring a man home to help perform the father's social obligations. When that happens, a father may have more opportunity to devote his time to affairs beyond his wife's family land, if he wishes.

Geffray (2000:14) explains that in a matrilineal kinship system in Iráti district of Nampula province, Pwiyamwene are important to understand gender relations. These are women who are placed in charge of ritual preparations within the family. Pwiyamwene are associated with land and conflict resolution. They are also influential in the raising of children, as a way to help young mothers fulfil their roles as mothers and women. In contrast, Medeiros (1985:22-23) argues that in the matrilineal kinship system in Nampula province, men could also be in charge of land with siblings. Medeiros shows changes in the ways gender relations have been understood in matrilineal kinship systems.

The patrilineal kinship system in southern Mozambique operates in the following way. Couples marry through lobolo, and thereafter live on the man's family land. In this system, marriages are less stable, and fertility is much more of a social issue; divorces occur due to infertility or suspected infertility of a wife. To prove that a man is fertile, the man's family often allows him to impregnate another woman. In some situations women are allowed to prove fertility, but for this to occur, the man's family must first accept that there is something wrong with their son; which is not likely to happen unless the family has previous experience of male infertility.

Junod (1996 [1927]:114-118) presents a detailed account of lobolo in southern Mozambique. He focuses on different stages families pass through to start and build a new family. Junod explains that lobolo practices have the effect of uniting men's and women's families and are relevant to fertility. Arnfred (2001:3) further describes some socio-political dimensions of lobolo practice during the period the revolution and the changes Frelimo made to lobolo after 1984.

The descriptions of matrilineal and patrilineal kinship systems are relevant in this discussion because they will help to understand the ways residents of

Mafalala barrio perceive sexual relationships, against the background of differing traditions.

Under the patrilineal kinship structure, there are definite double standards for sexual behaviour. It is clearly accepted that men can have more than one sexual partner or wife, and may have sex for pleasure; but women are only expected to have sex within the marriage and for procreation. Abortion and contraceptives are not encouraged and it seems that in such systems women enjoy little or no control over their reproduction. In this situation, a woman could be allowed to be impregnated by her husband's brother or nephew. In such a case, family members would expect the individuals concerned to keep the matter secret, although this is not always achieved — such things tend to come out when people are angry or get into conflicts with each other.

Despite the striking differences between the matrilineal and patrilineal kinship systems, there are also similarities in their attitudes to sex and sex roles. Men are expected to have sex with women, and sex is expected to involve penetration. Any other type of sexual relationship is not revealed or discussed. Men are expected to know everything about sex, while a woman's sexual preference or desire to know more tends to be ignored or silenced.

As a result of such taboos, women become adept at concealing their interest in sex and find it difficult to let their sexual desires and needs be known to their partner. Kinship practices will take time, perhaps generations, to change.

With regard to sexual education, some members of kinship networks, particularly the elders, have a responsibility to offer sexual and moral education to young people and to teach them about their gender roles. Some do this more effectively and sensitively than others. Elders also regulate the participation of each individual in the group; for example, they deal with matters such as wedding ceremonies, infertility treatment and divorce. In this way, gender roles become central in understanding individuals' responsibility within and outside the group.

In both matrilineal and patrilineal kinship systems, men are socialised to expect women to perform the roles of mother and wife, and women to perform these roles. On the other hand, women expect men to perform duties of husband and father, including protection and provision. Men who are unable to perform these roles do not regard themselves as committed to the woman concerned, as informants also made clear. Thus, gender and age of family members define each individual's position and role in the group. As they grow up, men are trained to be providers whereas women (especially younger women) are expected to be subordinate to the husband and family. A woman will typically have to wait until she is one of the elders of the family to exercise any form of leadership or wisdom role.

The discussion around the fragmentation of the family structure in Mozambique highlighted socio-cultural factors which influence some individuals to accept or reject the idea of 'safe sex'. This idea, though central to most HIV/AIDS awareness campaigns, has been criticised by scholars whose work has indicated the need to link local practices with condom use. These 'condom campaigns' have failed to analyse sexuality in a social context. As a result, there has been a failure to recognise that for some (perhaps many) individuals, their pre-existing beliefs, values and associations will prevent them from assimilating the concept of 'safe sex' in the intended way.

Having discussed the context of post-civil war Mozambique and the consequent fragmentation of the family structure, I will now provide a brief history of HIV/AIDS research in Mozambique.

A Brief History of HIV/AIDS Research in Mozambique

HIV/AIDS research has tended to rely on surveys to assess individuals' sexual behaviour. The search for the origin and causes (maintaining factors) of the HIV/AIDS pandemic has occupied the biomedical discourse. However, social science studies have shown the link between health promotion perspectives and societal responses to health issues (Falmer 1993; Stadler 2002; Weiss 1997). The beginning of HIV/AIDS research in Mozambique is not different from other countries of the world, in that this research has been based on the biomedical approach and has sought to discover the causes and cure or prevention of HIV infection.

The first diagnosis of HIV in Mozambique was made in the Cabo Delgado province in 1986. HIV was not regarded as a social problem because of the lack of knowledge about it. In any case, at the time of the first HIV diagnosis in the 1980s, Mozambique was a country embroiled in a civil war. The central focus of governmental and non-governmental organisations was to mobilise resources to help settle displaced people, and to provide food.

The Department of Epidemiology in the Ministry of Health (MoH) took responsibility for investigating the origin and spread of the disease in the country. Thus, in 1987 the MoH invited experts from the World Health Organisation (WHO) to elaborate a plan to deal with HIV. The WHO team conducted research that revealed six cases of HIV infection. However, they predicted that the HIV virus would spread in Mozambique due to its increased incidence in neighbouring countries, where the rates of infection were high. HIV was spreading through sexual intercourse (including heterosexual intercourse), blood transfusion, and materials exposed to infected blood — including traditional healers' use of non-sterile cutting objects, such as needles and razors.

At this stage, the spread of the HIV virus had two explanations. Firstly, there was the idea that promiscuity among prisoners during the civil war resulted in high rates of HIV infection. This meant rebel soldiers sleeping with women prisoners. This view produced a stigma around captured people, masking other routes of HIV infection, for example drug use. However, it was difficult to validate the idea of heterosexual promiscuity in camps because of the lack of documented records in the war-affected areas.

A less simplistic rationale holds that HIV increased because of the breakdown of family structures. People who lost (or were separated from) their families in the war, particularly children and youth, found it difficult to maintain family ties and values.

Secondly, the HIV/AIDS prevalence in the neighbouring countries and its spread to Mozambique motivated the MoH together with the WHO to draw up the National Programme against HIV (1988-1990). It was from this perspective that a programme was developed to train the first HIV educators in the country. The HIV educators were initially selected from health professionals employed by the MoH, although later on, community volunteers and members of NGOs were also trained as educators.

The MoH believes that information combined with knowledge about HIV infection and prevention could encourage individuals to change their sexual behaviour. This kind of intervention may have helped to keep HIV infections under control in some settings where individualism is a dominant social principle, but it did not produce effective results in Mozambique, where the origin and spread of the HIV have been explained without special attention to socio-cultural factors.

When the earlier HIV prevention campaigns were promoted in the country, the Ministry of Health team did not believe that HIV infections would stop. A major factor that undermined optimism at that time was the inability to gain access to rebel-occupied areas. Furthermore, the conceptions around health and illness held by the MoH and by ordinary people differed. Having already ignored the ways people understand health and illness in their explanations of HIV infections in Mozambique, the WHO and the Ministry of Health teams went on to build their HIV/AIDS awareness campaigns on the principle of individualism. Based on this principle, the AIDS campaigns appealed to individuals to change their behaviour by reducing the number of sexual partners and using condoms with occasional sexual partners. The targets of these messages were, in particular, commercial sex workers, truck drivers and displaced people.

The second phase of the NPA/HIV took place from 1990 to 1991. In this phase, the campaigns focussed on education and communication. In addition, the MoH invited Population Services International (PSI),[6] an American agency, to market condoms in Mozambique. PSI attempted to use the media, such as radio, television, newspapers and pamphlets (within and outside the MoH), to change the 'high risk sexual behaviour' of individuals. During this second phase, HIV/AIDS the main targets of prevention campaigns were youth, the military, and people already living with HIV/AIDS. In order to respond to social problems related to these target groups, the NPA/HIV started two research programmes, namely the biomedical and the social studies projects.

The biomedical studies focussed on the identification of more accurate technical interventions, laboratory diagnosis of HIV infections, transmission routes of the virus, and criteria for clinical diagnosis of HIV infections. These studies contributed toward the strengthening of the epidemiological understanding of the HIV epidemic, as well as identification of risk factors and co-factors for HIV 1 and HIV 2 infection; and the evaluation of treatment schemes for AIDS and opportunistic infections associated with it.

On the other hand, the social studies approach sought data regarding attitudes, sexual behaviour, knowledge and practices of individuals in different groups. The researchers looked at the receptiveness and interpretation of educational messages for the target groups. Research was also conducted on people's receptiveness to the NPA/HIV and its integration into the National Health Service system. Evaluation of counselling services for HIV-positive people and their families was another aspect of the social research undertaken at that time.

The culmination of the NPA/HIV was the production of the National Strategic Plan to Combat STDs, HIV and AIDS (2000-2002). The National Strategic Plan (NSP) was formed to monitor HIV/AIDS activities in the country. This plan has three main objectives. The first objective was to assess the extent of the HIV/AIDS epidemic. The second objective was to look at the national response to HIV/AIDS. This entailed the evaluation of health institutions and organisations working on the HIV/AIDS programmes in order to ascertain whether they were on track to help achieve the government's goals. The third objective of the NSP was to sustain the policy for three years. The current focus of the NSP was preventing HIV/AIDS infections among youth, especially girls, and sex workers. This goal rests on the assumption that girls and women were more vulnerable to HIV infection than boys or men. Simply because of the biology of sex, infected fluid remains in the vagina after the penis is withdrawn; and the female genital tract was lined with membranes, which provide less natural protection than the skin that covers the male penis.

This study aims to explore ideas about sexuality in a barrio of Maputo, called Mafalala, and relates these to the HIV prevention campaigns in Mozambique. Accordingly, the next section will present the history of Mafalala barrio, its people, and their coping strategies in the context of the diversity and complexity of everyday life.

The Mafalala Barrio

Geographically, the Mafalala barrio is located in the Urban District Number Three of Maputo City. Its total population at the time of study[7] was 21,189 inhabitants; of these 10,375 were men and 10,814 were women (INE 1998b). The barrio itself is bounded by the market of Adelina to the North, Marion Ngoabi Avenue to the South, Acordos de Lusaka Avenue to the West, and Angola Avenue to the East. There is a local perception that the barrio is composed of three Cells — A, B and C, and that it is subdivided into fifty-seven blocks.

Although the residents of Mafalala live in separate Cells, they meet for different purposes, such as going to church, going to the market, or visiting the mosque. The South-eastern area of the barrio is well served by infrastructure: there is easy access to the city, including the downtown areas, the commercial services centre and the industrial areas. The barrio is supplied with piped water, electricity and a telephone network, although these services are not available to all residents of Mafalala.

The Mafalala barrio was once known as 'Munhuana', meaning 'salt water' in the Ronga and Changana languages of Southern Mozambique, because the area was once below sea level. Because the soil still contains salt water, the land is not suited to agriculture. The name changed to Mafalala around the time that seamen from Mozambique Island (Nampula Province, in northern Mozambique) settled in this region: residents hold that the name Mafalala emerged from songs sung by these seamen on the weekends and during rituals of circumcision. Ritual tattooing and many sacrifices were regarded as feats of courage. Residents also said that the ritual was known as 'nífalala' or 'áfalala', meaning 'music and dance' in the Emakwa language.

According to Tivane (2002:16), three groups originally settled in Mafalala. The first of these groups were the Laurentinos: people born in Lourenço Marques, now known as Maputo. These were followed by traders from Mozambique Island and the Comoro Islands (the latter passing through Mafalala on their way to India to trade). The Comoro Islanders who settled in the barrio were also involved in the slave trade to the Americas. The third group, the Madjodojos, consisted of health professionals and musicians. Some people from the Madjodojos group lived in houses built from zinc and wood, which differentiated them from others in the barrio (Tivane 2002:15). This description is useful because it provides a picture of the diversity and complexity of the people living in the barrio.

After Mozambique's independence in 1975, the zinc and wood houses were nationalised. The Administração do Parque Imobiliário do Estado (APIE) rented out the houses for less than the South African equivalent of two rand per month. During my fieldwork, I heard from residents that they could not change the house structures because the government was planning to turn the barrio into a living museum. (However, in conversation with officials working in Mafalala barrio this information was not confirmed).

With regard to educational infrastructure, the barrio has two public schools which provide schooling from grade one to grade four. After grade four, pupils go to Escola Primária 25 de Setembro, Escola Primária da Munhuana, Escola Primária Estrela Vermelha and Escola Primária Noroeste 2. These primary schools are located within two kilometres of the barrio. Furthermore, children from barrios close to Mafalala, such as Xipamanine, Micadjuíne and Alto Maé, also attend Mafalala's public primary schools.

There is an official market called Adelina, and several garages in Cell A, as well as small services such as shops, hairdressers and repair shops. There is one police station in the Administrative Post of Mafalala barrio, and a small jail is attached to the Administrative Post. The jail is for so-called 'small offenses', such as stealing chickens or pick-pocketing. The barrio has also benefited from its proximity to Urban District Number One, particularly in terms of public services and access to the Central Hospital of Maputo. Nevertheless, when residents are sick, they seldom go to hospital because they have no money to pay for transport and medicines; instead, some go to traditional healers for treatment.

There is a strong religious following in Mafalala. In addition to Catholic churches, other Christian Churches represented include the Methodist Wesleyan Church in Mozambique; the Universal Kingdom of God, and the Twelve Apostles Church. There are also four mosques, each with its own name. The first is Braza, meaning 'the place of entertainment'. Cadria was named after the prophet and disciple Maome, and means 'the way to power'. Chadulia is named after another disciple, Ahmed Chadulia, and lastly, the name of the mosque Camararia means 'stone'. The Camararia mosque was later designated Itifaque which means 'agreement'. Chadulia is the largest mosque in the barrio, originally built by Muslims from Mozambique Island. Meanwhile, Muslims from Zanzibar, Comoro Islands and Tanzania created the Braza, Cadria and Camararia mosques (Lemos 1988, and Mussá 2001).

Whilst Mafalala contains a significant number of churches, it appears that Islam plays a prominent role in the barrio. It was notable that residents used the mosques for entertainment, to prepare weddings, and to organise funerals. The majority of residents using the services of the mosques had moved to Mafalala from different provinces. They could not afford to visit their families back home, so they have found the mosques useful. In mosques, residents were able to meet with people from their birthplace. They chat and reminisce about their 'home'. The mosques are also recommended by officials in Mafalala to researchers looking for centres of culture in the area.

After the end of the civil war many changes happened in Mafalala. People went looking for their relatives with whom they had lost contact during the war. Some informants learned that they had lost their family or members of their family. Others brought members of their families, or even entire families, to live in Mafalala, while some people who had enjoyed no previous links to the area took advantage of the situation and moved to there. As a result, the barrio is now overpopulated. The streets have become narrow, and many families comprise more than eight persons in a house, even though the houses are small and some have only two rooms.

The accommodation of new residents (internally displaced people) took place irregularly and spontaneously. For instance, new residents built houses in areas previously used for public space, such as the football field, utilising whatever free spaces they found without government control. The Mafalala land is not officially surveyed, a fact that also allowed for the emergence of new buildings everywhere. New buildings differed in quality from earlier buildings: while some were built of conventional materials such as bricks, cement and zinc, and were painted, others used non-conventional materials such as cardboard, poles and plywood. The new houses were often painted with mixed colours such as pink, purple, orange and yellow, since many residents could not afford to buy larger quantities of paint, but instead acquired leftover paints from informal markets. Due to overpopulation and irregular construction, the barrio has many footpaths but few streets wide enough for a car to pass. Moreover, paths are poorly lit, not for lack of electricity but because of vandalism. The greatest environmental problem, however, is soil impermeability. During the rainy season, there are always floods, which cause the overflow of pit toilets and destruction of wells. Therefore, in the rainy season diseases like malaria and cholera are common in the barrio. The lack of organisation among residents to keep drains clear also contributes significantly to the problem. With regard to cleaning the drainage, Guimarães (aged 32) says: 'We are not organised to clean the drainage. Some people do not take it seriously ... they start to clean the drainage when they see it is going to rain'.

The community centre of Mafalala barrio used to help clean the drains, but stopped due to a lack of cleaning resources such as dustpans, buckets and brooms. The coordinator of the community centre explained that previously the centre had sponsors, but that they now rely on contributions from the residents.

Having described the history of Mafalala barrio and some of the changes that have occurred over time, the next section will present the findings of my study about young people's perceptions of sexuality.

Perceptions of Sexuality

According to the Penguin Dictionary of Psychology (1987), the term 'sexuality' in English usage means something abstract, like 'sexual personality': 'All those aspects of one's constitution and one' behaviour that are related to sex ... the quality of being sexual'. In other words, sexuality refers to how a person expresses his or her sexual self, and includes attitudes and beliefs about sex. The term also conveys biological, emotional, and cognitive implications and is usually considered as something belonging to an individual rather than a group.

The responses of young residents of Mafalala barrio, however, do not suggest that they had the above concept in mind. Rather they describe 'sexual intercourse' or 'beliefs about sex' (as with César, and Eva, below).

Answering the question 'What is sexuality?', César says:

> Sexuality is normal because everyone does it. Sexuality is sexual intercourse between a man and a woman. – César, aged 23.

For César, sexuality is something that is obvious. In other words, there is actually no need to ask about sexuality because everybody knows what it is. César furthermore points to a definition of sexuality that is normative. For him, it is confined to sexual activity between a man and a woman. It is a 'natural' thing but also something that has social limits.

> Sexuality is sexual intercourse with girls of my age. I do not support adult men sleeping around with young people. This is because with young women adult men do not take responsibility for their actions. – Fernando, aged 21.

Fernando expects to have penetrative sex with 'girls' of his age, but also criticises adult men for wanting to do the same. This is because, in his view, adult men might not be responsible for the outcome. Fernando's comment calls attention to the existence of the so-called 'sugar daddies' in the barrio. These would perhaps correspond to the 'old, rich men' who were mentioned as possible victims of homosexual youth. From his point of view, the presence of the more affluent 'sugar daddy' makes it difficult to get girlfriends — he feels at a disadvantage. Fernando does not have enough income to 'tchunar'[8] a girlfriend and thus sees the 'sugar daddy' as a rival. His definition is less simplistic than Cesar's; if sexuality was only about what is 'natural', then the younger man would presumably have the advantage, but the wealth of the older man prevents this. For Fernando, sexuality is apparently very much about contest and prizes. He tries to level the 'playing field' with his claim that older men lack responsibility and that the girls are (by implication) only after their money.

However, Bento argues that:

> Sexuality is a biological cycle that begins when you are seventeen years old. It is an act that must be done between a man and a woman. — Bento, aged 22.

Bento argues that sexual activity must begin at seventeen. Bento associates sexuality with biological change. His account privileges procreation as the purpose of sexuality, and does not emphasise pleasure.

Such accounts fall outside the medical perspective, in which individuals are viewed primarily as biological entities, thereby neglecting the 'social field' in which they live. Medical discourses tend to universalise sexual practices that shape individual points of view. These discourses also sometimes explore individual symptoms in a way that facilitates stigmatisation of HIV-positive people. In this study, I am concerned with the meanings people give to sexuality precisely because they do sometimes embrace a different framework to that of the dominant medical discourse.

Having discussed young men's views of sexuality I will now turn to the young women's perceptions on the subject:

> Sexuality is a union of two people, a man and a woman. — Maria, aged 21.

Maria's argument shows that she understood sexuality as sexual intercourse. Maria also expects sexual activity to occur between heterosexual partners. I noted that Maria used the word 'union' to mean the sexual act. Perhaps this was to reduce embarrassment between Maria and the researcher.

Amélia explains that:

> [Sexuality] is a human necessity. Before, people said sex has an age. For instance, my grandmothers educated me not to have sex before I turned eighteen, but I know girls that began sexual intercourse at the age of thirteen. − Amélia, aged 20,

Amélia believes that the purpose of sexuality is procreation and it cannot be repressed. Her definition of sexuality suggests that the questions of biology and socio-cultural aspects are intertwined. This means that in situations where young women do not find a partner to marry, which is the kinship network's expectation, they may have a 'rider' − which gives individuals alternatives that are outside the control of the kinship network. In this sense Amélia understands sexuality to be for pleasure. Since Amélia received sexual education from her grandmother (by whom she felt protected), she feels sorry for girls who start sexual activity early. While the first two young women talked freely about sexuality, Eva simply stated:

> I do not know how to say ... Sexuality is linked with sex and pleasure. It must be done between man and woman. There are many ways of making sex. [I think] sex should be done with your own boyfriend. Girls that make sex with more than one partner are prostitutes. − Eva, aged 22.

Eva's response links biology with socio-cultural aspects. In this way, she associates sexuality with the sexual organs and their use for pleasure. Eva also highlights the fact that sexuality is something that happens between heterosexual partners, thereby demonstrating the legitimisation of sexuality discourses from Eva's point of view. Similarly Bertina asserts that:

> Sexuality has to do with sex after eighteen with your own boyfriend. When I have a boyfriend, I first study him to know if he really likes me. I then have sex with my boyfriend because I love and trust him. But I think that young people must have sex when they are twenty-eight because they will know how to care about themselves. At that age, they can work in any institution or set up business to improve their personal life. − Bertina, aged 20.

Bertina argues that love, trust and age are central issues pertaining to sexuality. It seems that Bertina views sexual activity as normal and acceptable once she has a boyfriend whom she can love and trust. Bertina's more individualistic attitude becomes evident when she talks about first 'studying' the boyfriend before having sex. It is interesting that she takes responsibility for deciding whether the man is suitable, although her comment about waiting until one is 28 — something she clearly did not do — suggests that perhaps there is also some insecurity or concern about the ability of younger women to 'care about themselves'. I would conjecture that Bertina associates the relationship with a boyfriend with sexual intercourse and personal benefit, rather than with family responsibility. Another young woman, Mariana, explains that:

> Sexuality is an act practised by two persons; I mean a man and a woman. It cannot happen among children but mainly with us young people. But I also know that there are young people that have sexual intercourse with people of the same sex, but that is wrong. — Mariana, aged 21.

Mariana showed that, in her view, sexuality is a youth activity, although parents are not expecting young people to be sexually active (see the explanation, below, of the expression 'cu kundzana'). Mariana criticises sexual activity among children, meaning that she does not approve of sexual intercourse among people that lack responsibility.

These arguments put forward by young women suggest that sexuality was mainly associated with physical contact and the biological function of sex. Sexuality is viewed as something given, and it is expected that one's sexuality is for the purpose of procreation. The question is: Can young people control sexuality? HIV/AIDS prevention campaigns are premised on the belief that individuals will change their behaviour if they know about the 'risk' involved and about health information. In emphasising the individual aspect of sexual activity in this way, the campaigns, however, fail to understand the socio-cultural context of sexuality or to consider that it is the socio-cultural context that constrains individuals' capability to act on health information. In the context of Mafalala, for instance, the socio-cultural is not only a constraint, but also an untapped resource. For example, grandparents are for many a useful source of advice on sexual behaviour. Many people decide to talk to their grandparents to find solutions for their intimate problems. It would be useful in stopping the spread of HIV/AIDS if prevention efforts could empower grandparents to help their younger family members.

I learned that the expression 'cu kundzana' refers to the sexual activity of married couples in southern Mozambique. It suggests that young, unmarried people are not expected to be sexually active. Yet the 'rider' situation, which I will discuss in the following section, indicates that young people are sexually active. One point that clearly emerges from the interview with younger women is that age is significant in their decision to start a sexual relationship, or at least to feel confident about doing so. Sexual activity, for them, appears to mean penetration. Kissing, hugging and sexual touching, for instance, were not features of the young people's everyday talk, suggesting that if these acts are part of usual sexual activity, they are not discussed.

Having described young people's views of their own sexuality, I will now turn to a discussion of dating and the 'rider'.

Dating and the 'Rider'

In the previous section, the 'rider' was identified as a casual or temporary sexual relationship, with no elements of commitment. There are many reasons young people start a 'rider relationship'. Fernando, for instance, explains how and why he starts a 'rider':

> I do not work but it does not mean that I cannot enjoy life. If I find a girlfriend she will need my attention ... It is not nice to have a girlfriend and not do tchunar[9] ... [a] 'rider' is practical and cheap. — Fernando aged 24.

During the fieldwork, young people used the word 'rider' to mean 'occasional relationship'. Fernando's idea about having a 'girlfriend' — a longer-term relationship — plainly includes the notion of providing economic support to him. To care about the girlfriend means to provide material things for her comfort. Fernando's view about a girlfriend and the way he would like to give her 'attention' indicates that Fernando does indeed wants to build a long-term relationship. Perhaps he is merely justifying his inability to commit to a relationship, but it is interesting to trace this assumption about 'girlfriends'. 'Rider', clearly, is a widespread practice but not necessarily the masculine ideal. Fernando has seen other young men able to 'tchunar' with their 'girlfriends' and wants to be able to do the same. Clearly, whatever his real reasons may be, Fernando is saying that he is not (yet) prepared to take on a long-term relationship; but he is also not planning to do without sex. This is where, from his point of view, the option of 'rider' becomes important.

I would say that Fernando is not only concerned about his ability to 'tchunar' his girlfriend because this is something he would like for himself. It seems likely that peer pressure is central to understanding Fernando's point of view. From that perspective, it is not difficult to understand Fernando's concern about his girlfriend's beauty: young people in the barrio are very much aware of fashion and appearance. At weekends, young men often walk around the barrio, in groups or alone, displaying. In doing so, they display themselves in fashionable clothes such as jeans, T-shirts, and caps with brand logos. The same behaviour occurs with young women, who wear jeans, mini-skirts, and tight dresses.

Clearly, it is important to Fernando to be seen as a (heterosexual) man. This might not necessarily involve sex, though; while the young people used the term 'rider' to describe an occasional sexual relationship, it was not clear whether 'rider' would always end in sexual intercourse. In the context of the above description of public display, Amélia's words may have a further significance:

> It is not difficult to find a 'rider'. You look at the way he looks at you, wears clothes and walk in the street. He will walk as if he is searching for something ... He will walk and ask you questions about someone else's address and he will say one word and another. If you are interested you will go with him. — Amélia, aged 20.

Amélia explains that the body movement was important to recognise a 'rider' (here, meaning 'sexually available young man'). Amélia also points to the relevance of clothes as sexual signals in this situation. Amelia's description of 'rider' associates body language and fashion with sexuality.

As stated previously, young men claimed that they frequently use condoms in 'rider' situations, and three young men in fact affirmed that they sometimes 'borrow' condoms from close friends on occasions where they lack the money to buy one, or find themselves in an unexpected opportunity to get a 'rider'. Concerning condom use, all the young men that I interviewed said that they prefer to use jeito,[10] a brand of condom that is perceived as lighter and thinner, as opposed to the MoH-issued condom. Nevertheless, there often were times when young men did not use jeito:

> When I have a 'rider' I know that I need jeito ... Sometimes, it is difficult to cope with the situation. I take a girl home to stay with me during the night and we need to make the cenas[11] but I am not sure if we cope to use jeito every time we do the cenas. — Riquito, aged 21.

Riquito's statement shows that despite his young age, he has taken a girlfriend home for sex. Riquito knows that he should be using condoms, but clearly is not doing so, at least some of the time. It is not clear what the reason for this might be, given his rather vague expression 'difficult to cope with the situation'. Riquito's statement does to some degree appear to evade being accountable for his sexual behaviour: it surely is not credible that a man would be unsure if he is wearing a condom or not.

It is surprising that young men talked more about condoms than young women did — even though women are more at risk of HIV than men. Perhaps young women are not expected to show their sexual preferences so clearly, but also the idea of trust is central to understanding young women's silence about sexual acts. As female informants made clear, 'trusting somebody' only happens in a long-term relationship. One can infer from this that in 'rider' situations where trust is absent, the women would prefer their partners to use condoms, but may not always be in a position to control that choice.

The 'rider' is not the only form of 'non-serious relationship' available to young people. It is also accepted that they may 'date', a casual form of relationship, which can be a preliminary to forming a long-term relationship. The purpose of such dating is for the couple to get to know each other, but it also involves having fun, the sharing of social life and (sometimes) having sex. As Fernando remarked, this kind of dating involves a lot of fashion, and there appears to be an expectation that 'boyfriends' will buy fashionable clothes and food for their 'girlfriends'.

Riquito and other young men knew about sexually transmitted infections, mainly syphilis and gonorrhoea. However, they only heard about HIV/AIDS infections on radio and television, and through public health initiatives. This suggests that there is as yet little or no 'local knowledge' of how to cope with the threats posed by HIV/AIDS. When infected by an STI, they know where to go for help, what to do and even the consequences of not treating these sexually transmitted infections properly. In this matter, young people mentioned that they have support from the adolescent and youth friends association. Despite the apparent social acceptance of (male) youth being sexually active, the young men say that when they become infected they would prefer go to hospital for treatment without informing their parents. Tito's experience suggests why this might be:

> When I realised that the martelo[12] was not fine, it was expelling a white flux. I told my brother. He advised me to tell my parents. After I told them they sent me to hospital but when I healed they joked about it. — Tito, aged 22.

Not surprisingly, Tito, who is still young and must have found this a painful and embarrassing experience, was uncomfortable with his parents' mocking attitude. Tito had expected his parents to keep the incident private.

As mentioned previously, the fact that Tito used the word 'martelo' to refer to his penis indicates that he considers himself a man. His embarrassment also suggests that he understands that this martelo problem was a sexual disease. However, this understanding is not always present among informants in Mafalala. Three young female informants spoke about friends who had become infected with syphilis and gonorrhoea, but their understanding or their claim was that hot weather and tight underpants had caused these diseases. This suggests that when young people encounter problems in sensitive aspects of their life they tend to externalise the reasons for their actions by shifting the blame.

It is interesting to note that even though ignorance about HIV and other STDs appears to be prevalent, some informants are aware of the effects of the disease on the community. For Eva, there is too much 'information' about HIV and not enough action to help infected people:

> We need medicine to help people living with HIV. It is not enough to inform people about the disease. I mean people are dying and it is important to find solutions to this problem. — Eva, aged 22.

Eva's argument is that providing information for young people is not enough. She is applying either/or logic — either information, or treatment. Yet people are also infected because of a lack of information, since they are not taking adequate steps to prevent becoming infected in the first place. This raises a critical question: What if Eva is part of the problem? What are youth themselves doing to prevent the spread of HIV/AIDS? What kind of knowledge do they have? Eva is one person who did have such knowledge; when interviewed, she was emotionally depressed because her neighbour died in December 2003, a victim of HIV/AIDS. Eva had also lost family members and friends to this disease. Yet she and her friends are not empowered to prevent infections among themselves.

Clearly many young women are not able to make their partners use condoms. They are also not absorbing sexual information from HIV/AIDS prevention campaigns because of socio-cultural practices. The condom campaigns that focus on the male usage of condoms separate sexual activity for procreation and pleasure. Condoms are available everywhere in the barrio, but as yet there has not been an adequate explanation or motivation which would help the youth to become more involved in the prevention campaigns, helping each other as they do with other social diseases.

Like Eva, Mariana (aged 21) is concerned about people living with HIV/AIDS. However, she reverts to a common misperception: poverty is to blame for the spread of the disease. People die because 'they do not have money to get medicines'. In Mariana's understanding, the illness exists but she does not understand what doctors (or medicines) can or cannot do to help AIDS patients; she does not understand that rich people can also die of the disease. Eva and Mariana are examples of urban youth who have only a partial understanding of the challenges posed to communities by HIV/AIDS. It seems likely that the youth in rural areas might have even less practical knowledge, since they have so little access to health services and communication.

It appears that for some young people at least, HIV/AIDS prevention campaigns have been successful in linking HIV, information and health, using the media to communicate health messages. But when these informants present solutions, the gaps in their knowledge of the disease become evident: both think actually that the problem is a lack of help and of treatment ('medicines'). As with many problems in their daily lives, they look at the situation through the lens of poverty and deprivation. In so doing, they may not be aware that everybody can be infected with the HIV/AIDS virus; nor that everybody can take steps to protect himself or herself, as long as they are willing to use condoms or able to ask their partner to use one.

Following this discussion of young people's perceptions about dating and the 'rider', I will now turn to their views about abortion.

Views on Abortion

According to the study's findings, it seems that young women are more concerned about abortion than young men are. This is because young men often seem to be able to evade responsibility for an unwanted baby. In any case, it appears that young men and young women have different attitudes towards pregnancy. Although pregnancy is also a way that allows young women to ensure that they are fertile, with regard to abortion Bertina and Maria revealed that women do sometimes seek voluntary abortions due to disappointment over their boyfriend's lack of willingness to accept or support the baby.

Three young women affirmed that they had had more than two voluntary abortions. These abortions were carried out at home with the assistance of close friends. Women would only go to hospital for treatment when they had a complicated abortion (retention of uterine contents).

Young women spoke about two kinds of abortions. The first kind of abortion is apparently performed with help from a close friend, while the other type of abortion, it is claimed, is made through drinking Coca-Cola mixed with Aspirin.[12] The first kind of abortion occurs as Maria explains:

> When I am sure that I am pregnant, for example, between two weeks to one month I tell my close friend. She waits until I am relaxed, and bites me on the back. The next day, my menstruation starts. — Maria, aged 21.

Maria believes that the biting in conjunction with the fear damages the foetus.

71

While Maria's description raises doubts about how seriously these women want abortions, it does demonstrate the importance of a close friend in her life, someone who is willing to share the burden and even the responsibility of ending the pregnancy.

Bertina describes the second kind of abortion:

> They [young women] put a bottle of Coca-Cola in the sun to heat up, and when it is hot, they drink it. Sometimes it is necessary to drink more than two cokes to cause an abortion. I heard that this kind of abortion is effective when the pregnancy is two weeks. — Bertina, aged 20.

Amélia, Bertina and Mariana believe that young men are not concerned about pregnancy because they see it as women's business. They feel free to assume that 'young women [the girlfriends] would only become pregnant if they wanted it'; this seems to be in line with Muanacha's assertion that a young woman might 'forget' to take her contraceptives if she wanted to fall pregnant. Yet clearly, the situation is far more complex than that. Sometimes young men do make token efforts to use jeito, and it is not clear that their female partner's preferences are being taken into account in the situation.

Although these young women talked about abortion, in general it remains a taboo topic, particularly among young women. Young women may expect to be sexually free, but they seem to lack even basic knowledge about their own bodies and their sexuality, and are not encouraged to learn more.

As we have seen from the foregoing discussion, young people's views on abortion and how they relate to fertility and sexuality can be problematic and sometimes unrealistic. The next section concludes this discussion.

Some Concluding Thoughts

This paper has provided an ethnographic approach to the perceptions of sexuality among young residents of Mafalala barrio. However, the results of this study should not be generalised to refer to the youth of Maputo in general, due to the complex and diverse background of these young people. The research can however be taken as a reflection of the issues currently faced by the youth with regard to sexuality and HIV/AIDS in contemporary Mozambique.

As discussed above, some of the young people's parents had after all moved from the war- affected areas of Mozambique to Mafalala barrio to seek better living conditions. Parents wished to see their sons and daughters married to a person that would respect their family's values. In this way, the family and the network represent protection and hope for young people that contrast with the idea of 'unsafe sex' based on interpretations propagated by medical clinics.

Young people seem to find themselves in situations where it is difficult to implement the idea of 'safe sex', partly because of peer pressure, but also because of family pressure to start and build a family of their own because of a lack of employment. These factors produced sexual relationships for pleasure (the so-called 'rider'). We have also seen that in the past, their experience of sexuality was rooted in the family context, in which sexual activity was for the purpose of procreation rather than for pleasure. In this sense, too, sexuality was associated with heterosexual partners and involved penetration.

In conclusion, then, I think that HIV/AIDS educational programmes seem to be ineffective due to uncertainty in the family about educational campaigns. For example, the original prohibition of local practices and their subsequent recognition left a gap in their children's education. Many families still use ritual initiations or advice from the elderly to educate their children about sex, sexuality and moral issues. Because of this gap, I suggest that HIV/AIDS educational programmes need to use the language of the family and work together with elders to capture their attention and to help to reduce the spread of HIV/AIDS virus in Mozambique.

Notes

1. At the period of the fieldwork José Bambo was final year student in Social Sciences at Eduardo Mondlane University in Maputo, Mozambique. He finished is course in 2005. His grandmother lives in the Mafalala barrio.
2. The official market located within the barrio.
3. 'Machaca' means family in the Ronga local language of Maputo. Through dance and music Machaca disseminates information about the HIV/Aids epidemic to youth living in and outside the barrio. Machaca has twenty-seven members and is attached to the Community Centre of Mafalala Barrio.
4. Timbila is a musical instrument similar to the piano, which produces a sound by using two sticks. It is considered world heritage by UNESCO since 2003.
5. At the time I was conducting this research, the Department of Social Anthropology at the University of Cape Town was debating the American Anthropologist Association's ethical issues.
6. The Population Services International is presently a National Non-governmental Organisation.
7. Tchunar' is slang to indicate someone who wears fashionable clothes.

8. The Population Services International wrote JeitO with capital 'J' and 'O'. In this paper I use the small letters for Jeito to mean a brand of condom advertised by the Population Services International.

9. Cenas is young people's slang for sexual intercourse. This word cannot be used between parents and children, but is only acceptable among young people.

10. Martelo means 'hammer'. It is a synonym for a man's penis in this context; this is contrasted to 'piriquito' which means 'lovebird' and is used for a boy's penis.

11. Although there is strong debate on abortion in Mozambique that has divided civil society into those one that would like it to be legalized and those that do not want it to legalized. The debate is around justice and human right issues (Artigo 358 do Código Penal).

12. I did not find any supporting data for this particular information. Nonetheless, it is clear that numerous abortions do occur in Mafalala.

Acknowledgements

The Council for Development in Social Science Research in Africa (CODESRIA) and the Social Science Research Council (SSRC) New York sponsored the research. Thank you so much to the many young residents of Mafalala barrio that kindly shared their experiences about relationships and sexuality. Thank you to Bambo, my research assistant and Eurico for proofreading. To Pérola, Ofélia and Sandra for informal discussion around youth and sexuality in Mozambique. The views and opinions expressed in this paper are those of the author and are not necessarily shared by the sponsoring organisations.

References

American Anthropological Association, 1971, 'Statement on Ethics', 'Principles of Professional Responsibility', *American Anthropologists Association*, AAA, available at http://www.aaanet.org/stmts/ethstmnt.htm.

Angrosino, M. and Pérez, K., 2000, 'Rethinking Observation: From Method to Context', in *Handbook of Qualitative Research*, pp. 673-701.

Arnfred, S., 2001, 'Family Forms and Gender Policies in Revolutionary Mozambique (1975- 1988)', available at http://www.cean.u-bourdeaux.fr/pubcean/td68-69.pdf.

Bernard, R., 1995, 'Participant Observation', in *Research Methods in Anthropology*, pp. 136-164, California: Alta Mira Press.

Caplan, P., ed., 2003, *The Ethics of Anthropology: Debates and Dilemmas*, London: Routledge.

De Queiroz, M., Demartini, Z., Cipriani, R., and Macioti, M., 1988, 'Experimentos com histórias de vida', in *Enciclopédia Aberta de Ciências Sociais*, pp. 2-43. São Paulo: Vértice.

Falmer, P., 1993, *AIDS and Accusation: Haiti and the Geography of Blame*, Berkeley: University of California Press.

Fortes, M., 1969, *The Web of Kinship*, Oxford: Oxford University Press.

Fox, R., 1967, *Kinship and Marriage: An Anthropological Perspective*, Harsmondsworth: Penguin Books.

Geffray, C., 2000, *Nem pai nem mãe: Uma rítica ao parentesco Macua*, Liboa: Ndjira/ Collecção Estudos Africanos.

Geração, Biz, 2001, *Fala menina..., fala rapaz... O manual do activista*, Maputo: Monaso.

Gillespie, S., 2000, *Beyond Kinship: Social and Material Reproduction in House Societies*, Philadelphia: University of Pennsylvania Press.

Goody, J., 1969, *Comparative Studies in Kinship*, London: Routledge and Kegan Paul.

Goody, J., 1973, *The Character of Kinship*, Cambridge: Cambridge University Press.

INE. Dez, 1998, *II Recenseamento geral da população e habitação (1997): Resultados definitivos*, cidade de Maputo, Maputo: Instituto Nacional de Estatísticas.

INE. Dez, 2001, *Inquérito nacional sobre saúde reprodutiva e comportamento sexual dos adolescentes e jovens*, INJAD, Maputo: INE.

INE. Dez, 2002, *Impacto demográfico do HIV/SIDA em Moçambique (actualização)*, Maputo: Governo de Moçambique.

Junod, H., 1996, [1927]. 'A significação inicial do lovolo e consequências', in *Usos e Costumes dos Bantus*, Tomo 1, pp. 114-118, Maputo: Arquivo Histórico de Moçambique.

Lemos, M., 1988, 'Reviver a ilha na Mafalala', in *Arquivo Histórico de Moçambique*, Maputo: Moçambique.

Medeiros, E., 1998, A representação da mulher nas estruturas do poder tradicional: O exemplo das sociedades do Norte de Moçambique, Maputo: Departamento de Arqueologia e Antropologia/UEM.

MoH, 2000-2002, *Plano estratégico nacional de combate as DTS/HIV/SIDA*, Maputo: Governo de Moçambique.

MoH, 1988-1990, *Programa nacional de combate ao SIDA*, Maputo: Governo de Moçambique.

MoH, 1990-1991, *Programa nacional de combate ao SIDA*, Maputo: Governo de Moçambique.

Mussá, F., 2001, 'Entre modernidade e tradição a comunidade islâmica de Maputo', in *Moçambique Ensaios*, pp. 111-133, Rio de Janeiro: UFRJ.

Nyamnjoh, F. B., 2007, 'Ethical Challenges and Responsibilities in Social Research: An Introductory Essay', in Apollo Rwomire and Francis B. Nyamnjoh, *Challenges and Responsibilities of Social Science Research in Africa*, Gaborone, OSSREA Botswana.

Paulo, M., 1998, 'Modernidade e Participação na sociedade Moçambicana: Uma contribuição para análise do fenómeno', *Estudos Moçambicanos*, Número Especial, Maputo: Centro de Estudos Africanos.

Paulo, M., 2003, 'Perceptions of HIV/AIDS in the Mafalala Barrio, Maputo, Mozambique', in Robin Cohen, ed., *Migration and Health in Southern Africa*, pp. 162-170, Cape Town: Van Schaik.

PSI, 2001, 'Mozambique and Marketing for AIDS Prevention III: Consumer profile Survey Report', Maputo: PSI/Mozambique.

PSI, 1999, 'Pré-testagem do Spot Radiofónico e do Panfleto Sobre o uso do Preservativo', Maputo: PSI/Moçambique.

PSI, 1998, 'Pré-testagem do Spot Televisivo e outros Materiais de Promoção', Maputo: PSI/Moçambique.

Reber, S., 1987, *The Penguin Dictionary of Psychology*, p. 694, London: Penguin.

Stadler, J., 2002, 'Rumour, Gossip and Blame: The Cultural Production of AIDS in a Lowveld Village', Pretoria/Reproductive Health Research, Paper presented to the Association for Anthropology in Southern Africa.

Thomas, W. and Znaniecki, F., 1958, *The Polish Peasant in Europe and America*, New York: Dover Publications.

Tierney, W., 2000, 'Undaunted Challenge: Life History and the Postmodern Challenge', in *Handbook of Qualitative Research*, pp. 537-553, Thousand Oaks: Sage Publications, Inc.

Tivane, D., 2002, 'Mafalala o poço das mil e uma histórias', pp. 15-16, Revista Proler, Número Especial, Maputo: Moçambique.

Weiss, M., 1997, 'Signifying the Pandemics: Metaphors of AIDS, Cancer and Heart Disease', *Medical Anthropology*, 11 (4), pp. 456-476.

Wyn, J. and White, R., 1995, 'The Concept of Youth', in *Rethinking Youth*, pp. 9-14, London, Sage Publications.

Of Perfumed Lotions, Biscuits and Condoms: Youth, Femininity, Sexuality and HIV and AIDS Prevention in Rural Gwanda District, Zimbabwe

Rekopantswe Mate

Introduction

Globally, the AIDS epidemic as a largely sexually transmitted condition has put the spotlight on sex in unprecedented ways. Social scientists have called for a focus on sexuality (Pollak 1992) as a way of understanding the complex bundle of socially accepted beliefs, myths, attitudes, norms and behaviours about sexual acts, one's role in them and behaviour towards the same and opposite sex (Varga 1997, also Van Eeuwijk and Mlanga 1997). Sexuality is closely connected to gender socialisation, ideals of femininity and masculinity, or notions of 'proper' male and female behaviour but is also textured by the socio-economic environment in which the relations occur. Consequently, sexual acts and beliefs about what is appropriate do not occur in a social vacuum.

HIV and AIDS prevention discourses generally decry 'culture' or 'tradition' as hindrances to behaviour change, echoing ethnocentric debates about culture and tradition as a hindrance to 'modernisation' and social change (Goldthorpe 1983). Often commentators do not acknowledge the role of notions of modernity at the margin as a risk factor and that instead of referring of 'culture' and 'tradition' as frozen in time there is in fact hybridisation (Holton 1998) of local ways of life as people internalise or devise new ways of life in response to a variety of pressures. Current public health messages connected to HIV and AIDS prevention tend to be a one-size-fit-all and ready-to-use list of dos and don'ts[1] (Kaler 2003). At grassroots level they are reinterpreted and adjusted to the disparate local situations in which they are consumed (Barnett and Whiteside 2002). Awareness and use of these messages are supposedly linked. The awareness, sometimes referred as 'knowledge', is erroneously measured through Knowledge, Attitude,

Practice and Behaviour (KAPB) surveys which invariably find that there is a high awareness of what HIV is, how it is transmitted and is preventable because people are parroting the ABCDs (which have now stretched to G) of prevention. That is, KAPB surveys ask 'status quo questions' to which 'status quo answers' are given (Crewe 2004). The 'knowledge' thus gathered does not seem consistently to inform behaviour. Consequently, lived realities are floating somewhere out there unseen, neither dealt with by interventions nor captured by surveys. This incongruence between knowledge as seen in KAPB survey responses and behaviour on the ground may be seen as 'irrationality' on the part of affected populations (Dilger 2001). In reality, it challenges the assumptions on which public health models of HIV and AIDS prevention are based. That is, the assumption that once people have information and knowledge or are aware of disease causing factors, they are likely to use the information to respond to a threatening situation such as the risk of HIV and AIDS. Justifiably these concerns have increased the need to understand human sexuality. In other words, the ABCDs of prevention do not exist and cannot work in a social vacuum. An understanding of socio-cultural circumstances in which people have sex allow us to understand how the ABCDs are reworked to suit prevailing pressures at the local level.

This paper is based on a research project that sought an understanding of discourses of youth[2] sexuality in rural Zimbabwe from both youths' and parents or guardians' perspectives. The paper focuses only on female youths and argues that they deploy their sexuality and femininity to access modern goods such as biscuits, fizzy drinks, and perfumed lotions in a bid to be 'with the world' (Friedman 1996) in a context in which they are otherwise marginalised and where these commodities are not accessible. The paper argues that the means by which these youths access these commodities constitute a reworking of prevailing local norms of dating and understandings of proper male and female roles leading to social-sexual exchanges between men and women of different ages. On one hand, the obvious socioeconomic inequalities between the parties limit possibilities of the use of condoms in spite of knowledge about HIV and AIDS, how it spreads and how it can be prevented. On the other hand, the gendered needs of either party (for men, the quest for sex with young women symbolises virility, spending on them symbolises economic prowess, and the search for marriageable partners; for women: the need for goods and services accessible with money they do not have and also the search for marriageable partners) seem to make it impossible for safe sex to be practised.

Youths and Youth Sexuality: Implications of Competing Views, Expectations in Zimbabwe

It is widely accepted that most HIV infections in Southern Africa in general occur during the onset of adolescence and among young adults or from teens to the early twenties (see Simbayi et al., 2004; Langhaug et al., 2003), as seen in the considerable upsurge of infection rates from age 14/15 years up to 24 years. This points to unsafe sex. In most societies this is alarming as it threatens future generations. However how best to respond to the sexual needs and challenges of youths seems closely connected to normative notions of their sexuality pitted against scientific, western medical views on how to deal with the public health threats implied by such practice

In contemporary non-western societies youths are defined on the basis of relational considerations as opposed to the use of age which is prevalent in western definitions. Bledsoe and Cohen (1993) note that 'youth' denotes being junior and that there are gradations of being junior which change with one's life cycle. Thus anyone can be defined as a youth depending on the situation. Youths defer to elders and ideally follow their instructions. Youth sexuality is not distinct in this situation, but like all other sexualities is bound by the principle of legitimacy of social relations in which sex occurs. Marriage is ideally the forum within which people have sex, in which case concerns of age are not important as long as the relationship is approved of within the cultural setting (Bledsoe and Cohen 1993). This is not to say that there is no notion of age of sexual consent but that adolescence in some sense signals marriageability as far as it points to reproductive abilities. Otherwise unmarried youths should not have sex, as this is considered socially disruptive even though it is increasingly common.

Principles of premarital chastity do not apply similarly to male and female youths. Female adolescence is generally underlined by restricted mobility and tight surveillance in a bid to control female sexuality and fertility, while male youths live through their adolescence without much parental supervision and control (Baylies and Bujra 2000, Bledsoe and Cohen 1993, see also Dowsett et al., 1998). Yet male virility persists as proof of masculinity. Women who behave like men in this respect are likely to be described as 'loose' (Dowsett et al., 1998, Katapa 1998). This is because in non-western societies family honour continues to hinge on notions of female virtue and uprightness linked to so-called virginal chastity (Fuglesang 1994). In patrilineal bride wealth systems as practised in Zimbabwe, virgins theoretically fetch a higher bride wealth thereby affirming family honour. Practically, in contemporary Zimbabwe virginity is usually hard to prove[3] in the absence of ceremonies celebrating the consummation of marriage, as practised in the past, in which virginity tests were performed and virgin brides celebrated and non-virgins humiliated. Still, the values of virginal chastity persist, in the form of expectations of females shunning sex outside and before marriage. In reality young women do have sex with unmarried and married partners for a variety of reasons including the need for intimacy and socio-economic factors (see Baylies et al., 1999; Bond 1997; Schoepf 1995; Kaler 2003; Dover 2002; Nyanzi et al., 2000). Nonetheless, female youths cannot flaunt their premarital sex escapades without the social costs of labelling and ostracism (Van Eeuwijk and Mlanga 1997; Kutapa 1998; Dowsett etal. 1998).

In the past, expectations of sexual abstinence outside and before marriage were supported by a complex web of institutions endowed with monitoring systems and means of controlling people of all ages and statuses (see Ahlberg 1994; Halle-Valle 1999). In some societies non-penetrative sex was an accepted practice among youths — anecdotal reports show that some of these practices were prevalent in the past in the area of study. Colonial experiences and Christianity destroyed these institutions and left only values that seem hard to live by given changed circumstances and the absence of commensurate institutional and living arrangements. Now sex has been simplified to penile-vaginal sex and is ideally out of bounds for all people who are not married — hence the A of the ABCs (see Marindo et al., 2003). Still, in spite of these changes, notions of an ideal past persist and permeate policies and debates on youth sexuality. The idea that youths are 'a window of hope' in the fight against HIV and AIDS seems to have intensified the quest to use 'traditional' methods, such as virginiy testing (see Scorgie 2002). Past norms and practices of non-penetrative sex have been forgotten.

Non-western views of youths and youth sexuality co-exist with western ones which are influenced by a variety of ideological and professional approaches, not least feminism, and medical and legal professions as seen in the work of multilateral organizations such as the UN. In the work of these organisations, youths are defined in terms of age, which is a proxy for physiological development (Simbayi et al., 2004). Concern with youth sexuality is connected to the well-being of the individual as well as concern with rights connected to reproductive health, namely the right to information about diseases of and transmitted through the reproductive tract and/or sex, how to prevent them and where to get treatment. In this case, youth sex, especially when it occurs in early teens, is seen as a threat to physiological development particularly if it leads to unplanned pregnancy, infection by a Sexually Transmitted Infection (STI) or HIV. Given HIV and AIDS, all individuals have to be informed to protect themselves and contraceptives made available to prevent unwanted pregnancies and diseases. This remains a challenge in a context where youths are idealised as 'asexual' by their families and communities.

In Zimbabwe the western perspective has internal contradictions. For instance the age of sexual consent is sixteen, meaning that an individual below that age seeking contraception is engaging in illicit behaviour in which the older partner is likely to be tried for statutory rape (see Langhaug et al., 2003). Add to this the fact that feminist views on teenage sexuality (which influence the debate on the rights of women and girls to reproductive health) in Africa tend to see girls and (young) women as victims of predatory male sexuality and patriarchal constructions of femininity, it is clear that there is confusion as to how to manage female youth sexuality. In spite of talk of empowerment, female youth sexuality is not yet a matter for celebration.[4] While one cannot deny that there is an element of abuse and exploitation in inter-generational sex, this view plays down the fact that girls and young women also actively explore their emerging sexuality and femininity (McRobbie 1991) and as such have social agency in their sexuality. However, this agency is experienced within social relations in which it is not acknowledged. Acknowledging it stigmatises women, who are ideally passive beings. In reality female youths are not and should not be seen as asexual, naïve beings whose participation in sexual relations is at all times as passive partners. That is, female youths actively deploy their sexuality albeit within understood local norms which they manipulate. As this paper will try to show female youths have internalised some notions of traditional expectations but have to contend with current realities and pressures. Thus given changing socioeconomic circumstances, 'traditional' expectations are hard to live up to and their realisation seems to be an obstacle course that has to be navigated with extreme caution, often without the wherewithal for a successful expedition.

Socio-economic Aspects of Sexuality

It has been noted that marriage remains the ideal institution in which people should have sex. It is (as was the case in the past) initiated and maintained through the exchange of material and non-material goods between partners and their families (Baylies et al., 1999; Dover 2002; Weiss 1993; Baylies and Bujra 2000; Halle-Valle 1999; Nelson 1987). In the past, the goods that were exchanged were symbolic and signified commitment and cemented new-found affinal relations. The role of gift exchange as the glue that holds relations together has been transformed by complex colonial histories and legacies combined with the prevailing circumstances of poverty and 'the logic of the market' (Ugarteche

2000). The latter is underlined by competitive relations between people, envy, and an understanding that one's needs are only met if one has access to cash (Ugarteche 2000). In view of poverty and desperation, people do not shy away from selling sex. Thus whereas in the past sex and sexuality were useful as part of forming alliances, sexual activity may now be for personal gratification (Foucault 1978) and personal power games and gains. Increasingly, transient sexual relations (as opposed to marital ones) are the basis of the exchange of goods. This has become the basis of economic security for individual women, and for individual men it brings power over women. This has created a situation where differences between and among wives, girlfriends, mistresses and commercial sex workers are not so clear (Dover 2002; Baylies and Bujra 2000). Women move easily between these statuses that mark different means by which they relate to and access resources from men (Halle-Valle 1999). For (young) men with no resources, marriage and parenthood are insurmountable expenses so they settle for other relations with women — girlfriends and commercial sex workers (Kutapa 1998; Mate 2005b; Bledsoe and Cohen 1993) while rich men can afford all four and the economic redistribution they entail. In turn, many women give birth out of wedlock and many while they are in their teens because the envisaged marriages fail to materialise. Elders in non-western societies are generally concerned about this type of sex (and the sexuality surrounding it) . Confronted now by HIV and AIDS, they attribute the scourge to this sexual behaviour and the failure of young women to restrain themselves in accord with traditional expectations.

The Research Setting

This study took place in two wards[5] (wards 12 and 17) of Gwanda district, which is situated in Matabeleland South province, on the south-western recess of Zimbabwe bordering Botswana. The population of the two wards is predominantly Sotho-speaking, although Ndebele is largely the lingua franca in commerce and public interaction (including in schools). Economically, Gwanda like the whole province is a low rainfall, chronically food deficit region. The successive 'below normal' rainy seasons since 1999 have compromised food stocks at household levels and unleashed what donor agencies have termed a 'humanitarian crisis', not only in the district but the whole of southern Africa. The district has insignificant manufacturing industries. It relies more on primary industry in the form of game and beef ranches, some of which have since closed in the wake of the 'fast track land reform' programme; and a few gold mines, some of which have either closed or scaled down operations in response to declining world prices of gold. Due to proximity to South Africa and Botswana, short and long term migration have become livelihood strategies of choice in the district, and especially in these wards (see Zinyama 2000). Of late however migration has become difficult, although not impossible, as the Botswana and South African authorities have taken to mass deportations of Zimbabweans suspected of being illegal immigrants.

Those who cannot migrate make a living through alluvial gold panning and small-scale gold mining, albeit using simple technology. Gold panning is associated with higher disposable income that is often spent very rapidly on personal leisure. It is a favourite local odd job, ahead of cattle herding, domestic work and piecework such as fencing fields, harvesting and so on. Its popularity has seen men and women (including youths) leave their homes to set up temporary camps for months on end on river banks and at disused mine shafts. Some youths start gold panning as a means of raising money for school fees and end up quitting school altogether. There are people who come from other towns to sell provisions at inflated prices and others come to buy gold. Some gold panners and miners send remittances and goods to those left at home.

Generally, gold panning is said to be socially and ecologically disruptive. Relations between men and women have changed as income-earning women and children no longer accept traditional norms of subordination. The proliferation of this activity is associated with increased commercial sex work, crime, and more generally a greater unruliness among young men. Ecologically, the panners leave gaping holes in the ground which become death traps for livestock. They increase the likelihood of poisoning water with the cyanide they use to process gold. Due to remittances from small-scale gold mining, from migrants and cross-border traders, province-wide levels of household income are actually comparatively high (IDS-UNDP 2003). Thus despite poverty, emergent survival strategies such as mining and migration have also altered consumption patterns. There is a preference for imported goods (footwear, clothes, accessories, toiletries and so on) from Botswana, South Africa and Zambia to some extent. Most clothing appanels are from Chinese manufacturers imported through complex migrant networks.

Methodology and Research Methods

This study used several methods, both qualitative and quantitative, although this paper relies on the qualitative aspects of the study. Some people polled in the quantitative survey joined the focus group discussion (FGD). Issues in the quantitative survey were similar to the ones on the FGD checklist and to the issues discussed with key informants. The quantitative survey is not incorporated in this study because in retrospect it was based on what Mary Crewe (2004) describes as 'status quo questions' to which 'status quo' answers were given. The survey sought to establish youths' knowledge and awareness of STIs, HIV and AIDS and their prevention, and youths' understandings of adolescence, preferred traits of ideal marriage partners, etc. Because of the one-to-one nature of the interviews, few female youths admitted to 'ever having sex', except for those with children. In FGDs a different picture emerged in which sex involving female youths with their male peers or older men is reportedly common. This was corroborated by older persons (parents and guardians in FGDs and as key informants. Thus qualitative methods are ideal for studies on sexuality because they allow researchers to understand the contextual aspects of sexuality (Varga 1997). In FGDs youths had an opportunity to explain the variance between 'knowledge' and 'awareness' of HIV and AIDS, and the difficulty of putting prevention messages to use. FGDs are especially suited for sexuality research because they enable social interaction and collective analysis of group concerns, information, knowledge and practices (Kitzinger 1994: 159–166; Dowsett et al., 1998). Researchers are able to probe group concerns and norms, shared experiences and attitudes which come out in the form of jokes, innuendoes, slips of the tongue, satire and non-verbal communication (exchanged looks, giggles etc.,) which can be withheld in a one-to-one interview. A limitation might be that some of this innuendo might be missed by researchers, who are invariably out-siders in the moral community of the people they are researching. In addition, although there were numerous occasions when we (participants and I) laughed as I listen to the recorded conversations, I wonder if we were laughing at the same thing. One is unfortunately not always able to capture, in writing, the atmosphere in the FGD in order to show the extent of perceived mutual understang which prevailed during the discussion.

In each of the two wards there were three meeting places, but in the end only five sites were visited.[6] A total of eleven single-sex youth and four mixed-sex adult FGDs took place. Discussions were facilitated by the principal researcher in local languages, namely SiNdebele laced with Sotho. The discussions were recorded on a micro-cassette recorder (nine and a half hours of discussion) and later transcribed verbatim by a colleague in the African Languages Department, leading to over 200 pages of transcriptions. Asking someone to transcribe the tapes allowed me some critical distance from the data for a while and made it easier for me to read through and translate the transcriptions into English. Data analysis was based on thematic concerns which arose in the discussion, in part prompted by the checklist of issues I had developed beforehand as indicated above. Discussions were conducted in such a way that a natural flow of issues was allowed. The similarity of issues raised by youths in different locations meant that I had reached a 'point of saturation' — that is, a point at which the number of FGDs would no longer add any qualitative difference to the data gathered.

At the end of the FGDs youths were invited to ask questions on issues related to the discussion which were unclear to them. These questions were very interesting to reflect on later as an indication of prevailing understandings of safe sex vis-à-vis HIV and AIDS (see Chikovore et al., 2002). I tried to answer them as simply as I could. The questions focussed mostly on the safety of condoms. Some wanted to see a female condom and asked how women use it. Others wanted more information on signs and symptoms of STI infections for men and for women. Youths with children also asked about cervical cancer and the effect of using herbal suppositories and douches to heighten sexual pleasure. On the question of condom efficacy I could only explain theoretically since I had neither condoms on me nor dummies on which to demonstrate their use. This was a shortcoming that had not been foreseen. Generally, one gets the impression that youths are concerned with broad issues of reproductive health and have information gaps and misconceptions.

Findings of the Study

Generally, female youths are aware of HIV and AIDS and how they are spread, and yet they are also acutely aware of local social and personal circumstances of poverty, emerging livelihood strategies and socialisation which together push them towards behaviours that are not prudent in the context prevaiing HIV/ AIDS prevention messages.

Understandings of Adolescence, Dating and Sex

Although in the literature there is an erroneous belief that there is no notion of adolescence in Zimbabwe (see Langhaug et al., 2003), it is not the case in all Zimbabwean cultures. In the study area, respondents refer to the onset of adolescence as 'ukuthomba' which in siNdebele refers to the time when both girls and boys show signs of physiological change. Alternatively in everyday talk people may refer to it as 'ukukhula', literally meaning 'growing up'. Beyond the physiological changes respondents also reported that there are behavioural aspects such as dating or being more aware of the opposite sex. Females reportedly become more conscious of personal adornment and deportment. Female respondents in this study said that all other physiological signs of growing up come without much fanfare except for menstruation, which must be communicated to older female members of the family such as the father's sister, older sisters, grandmothers but never one's mother as a sign of respect. The person to whom the matter is reported informs the girl's mother who tells the girl's paternal aunt (father's sister) who in turn formally tells the girl's father.[7]

The onset of menstruation is communicated to the family because the patrilineage has an interest in the reproductive abilities of its daughters. Besides menstruation has budgetary implications these days in the form of modern sanitary ware. Because most adolescents are generally without independent income, they cannot access sanitary ware without telling their parents or guardians.[8] When asked how older female relatives impart information to the girls, responses were vague. For instance, the relatives reportedly say 'Do not play with small girls, as they are not discreet if you soil your clothes while menstruating'.

Although not playing with small girls is supposed to show that the girl is now a 'grown up' and different from little girls, adolescent girls do not necessarily have license to behave as they please. Relatives apparently emphasise the need to avoid male company. They say 'Do not let boys touch you... Do not play with boys ... Don't let boys touch your breasts; it gives the wrong sensations, which might lead you to doing wrong things. If a boy touches your breast you get feelings you cannot control.

Asked whether boys in fact do fondle girls' breasts, the girls generally confirm that unsolicited fondling does take place. As for the 'wrong' sensations leading to 'wrong things', it was explained that this is sex. In a television talk show[9] which aired on 4 June 2005, a participant emphasised that girls must be told not to let boys touch them even on the shoulder because it leads to touching elsewhere and eventually leads to illicit sex. In the FGDs girls also said they are told 'to be respectful' ('ukuhlonipha' or 'ukuba lembeko') of older persons and males especially, presumably to avoid inter-generational sex. The 'respect' implied here includes respecting rules and norms of avoidance and the maintenance of social distance in order to be inaccessible to older members of the opposite sex. Thus from the onset of adolescence girls are socialised to shun male company and not to be keen on sex.

Despite these vague moral lectures about avoiding male company in general but also intimate male company, dating and premarital sex are reportedly very common, including relations with older males. Female youths dating is seen as an inevitable precursor to marriage and allows young men and women to choose and test the suitability of future marriage partners. Respondents explained that parents and guardians' lectures should not be taken literally because they (parents and guardians) also expect marriage from the girls. Until a marriage proposal is made boyfriends are for 'fun', 'recreation', ('ukuzilibazisa'), 'companionship and friendship' ('ubungani'), for managing loneliness ('ukuqeda isizungu') and also as a form of social security for girls from poor families in the form of gifts in cash and in kind that are exchanged in the relationship.

Female youths indicated that gifts are a sign of love and commitment in a relationship. The frequency of gift-giving and the value of gifts indicate a male partner's generosity and are a proxy for his ability to provide in marriage. Girls explained that their parents do not expect them to get married to men who cannot provide for them, hence these assumptions. Primarily the man has to have income to pay bride wealth, usually several head of cattle or the cash equivalent. In this vein, men with income such as gold panners, rural-based civil servants, including teachers, bus crews, returning migrants and others are attractive potential boyfriends. The girls indicated that even when a boyfriend is of limited economic means he has 'to make an effort' and find an odd job (such as fencing someone's fields, herding other people's cattle, gold panning etc.,) or save his pocket money if he is a schoolboy in order to give his girlfriend.[10]

Gifts that are received from boyfriends are in the form of cash which is used for personal expenses such as buying snacks, but the money might be squirrelled away and allowed to accumulate so that the recipient is able to buy toiletries including sanitary ware or items of underwear. Greetings cards such as Valentines, Christmas, birthday and general cards with romantic messages were also mentioned as possible gifts that are given or expected. Sometimes couples exchange personal photos which in a rural setting are quite expensive.[11]

Reciprocity whether balanced or generalised is essential to sustain gift exchange and cement the commitment in a relationship. Thus girls too are obliged to give gifts to acknowledge their appreciation of attention from and the 'commitment' of a male partner. They too give in cash and/or kind. Asked about sources of money, out of school youths indicated that they do odd jobs including gardening, doing housework for better off households or saving some of the money they get from boyfriends. Sex was also mentioned as a gift that is most available albeit one that should not be given easily as this might lead to the girl being seen as 'easy' or 'loose'.

Sex as a gift roused animated debate in all FGDs with male and female youths giving the impression it is an essential element of the social exchange in male-female relations, but debated the terms and circumstances surrounding girl's consent to sex. One female FGD participant said that relationships '... these days ... are about sex. Boys fall in love for sex'. This was countered by someone who said that '... If you let a boy lead you on, of course, sex is inevitable', and another who said 'Most girls get into relationships knowing that eventually there will be sex' and that 'Boys cheat girls. If a girl comes from a poor family a guy can help her with money but only if there is sex'. These debates show that female youths do have sex despite elders' lectures not to and that the sex is had in the process of trying to secure relationships in order to ensure marriage. However sex is sometimes agreed to because receiving a gift invariably obliges one to reciprocate and failure to do so is seen a sign of deviance, greed and manipulativeness. It is a sign of impropriety (see also Dover 2002); an unbalanced exchange and therefore not fair. In the local lingua franca, siNdebele, this is described 'ukudla umuntu', literally this means 'eating a person' but it suggests spending someone's money using uncouth means; spending money which one is not otherwise entitled to, taking advantage of someone or cheating. Only loose women and commercial sex workers are associated with this behaviour. Men and boys do not want to be 'eaten' in this way so they try to get their gifts' worth and more if the girls are not so astute. Thus in spite of its 'illicitness', youth sex also revolves around notions of propriety and fairness. Below is an excerpt on sex and gifts from two FGDs held in ward 17 (Bengo and Fumukwe on 28 and 27 April 2004 respectively).

RM: So once a guy gives a gift a girl has to agree to sex?
- If she wants to avoid a beating, yes. [Laughter from other participants]
RM: Are you sure that one risks a beating for saying no to sex after receiving gifts?
- Ye-es [in unison]
[One person speaks] — Actually, some girls are eager for sex not just to appease their boyfriends; but to pre-empt beatings.
- Some seem eager out of fear of beating.
- You get beaten because the guy is afraid that you have another boyfriend with whom you are having sex and hence you refuse to have it with him yet you are taking advantage of his money ('ukumudla').
RM: Do girls agree to sex as a sign of fidelity then?
- There is no other way, yes.
RM: No other way ... what do you mean?
- [Previous speaker] I mean you cannot say no, can you?
- You can.

- You can say no by saying that you cannot have sex with him but would rather wait.

RM: Do you then indicate a time limit?

- [Previous speaker] Not really. The point is if he cannot wait he can find another girl who is willing to have sex.

- You have not been beaten up that's all.

- If you've spent his money then he is entitled to a [cash] refund if you cannot have sex.

- Why accept his money or gifts if you want to say no to sex?

- But do we date so we can have sex? I do not think so? [She laughs and so do others]

- I think [sounding hesitant] ... the sex is for mutual enjoyment or fun ('ukukholisa'). — Bengo girls, 28 April 2004.

At another meeting place the previous day, following a discussion on the feasibility of abstinence, here is what youths said about why some youths have sex.

RM: Why the sex then? Why can't both of you wait?

- The sex keeps the relationship going (said with laughter with the rest of the participants also responding with laughter).

- If you are in a relationship, sex is par for the course. Otherwise why get in it in the first place?

- Sex is to enable us to get married.

- Sex is to get money for lunch while at school.

RM: Don't your parents give you money for lunch or can't you get a packed lunch from home?[12]

- They [parents] do not give us money.

- Parents give you a little bit [of money] sometimes, enough to buy a freezit,[13] but maybe I want a small packet of biscuits or sweets.

RM: So do you get the money by having sex?

- Look, you cannot spend a guy's money for nothing. You have to have sex with him.

- No it is not true if he really loves you he will give you money for nothing in return.

- Without sex? Impossible!!

89

[Animated and inaudible debate among participants].
- Yes, that is rare. You cannot spend a man's money for nothing. If you spend the money it is obvious you will have sex with him — Fumukwe girls, 27 April 2004.

In other words just as girls said that boys cannot make excuses for not giving presents by saying that they are 'too poor' to get money for a gift, girls cannot make excuses about being 'unable' to reciprocate because sex is in a sense potentially available to all people at all times. As parents in ward 12 noted, some girls have several boyfriends to maximize gift receipts which leads to confusion in the event of a pregnancy. This increases the likelihood of single parenthood; a situation which puts pressure on their parents' already meagre resources. Thus possibilities of marriage are squashed by entrepreneurial dating.

On the girl's part, it seems once she has a boyfriend, saying no to sex after receiving gifts is an uphill struggle. If she is not willing to have sex, her consent can be wrung out of her through manipulation, peer pressure, threats of or real force. Girls' reluctance to have sex is connected to real concerns about falling pregnant. Gifts compromise girls' ability to say no to sex and yet they are a sign of love and an indicator of whether or not a man is marriageable, that is, will he be able to provide for a family. How females deal with gifts from men seems to define 'decency' and 'fairness'. Girls who accept gifts and cannot reciprocate with the 'ideal' gift of sex are seen as greedy and wayward. A beating from a boyfriend seems justified as indicated in the excerpt above. The only way to avoid this dilemma is to avoid being in a relationship in the first place, but this forecloses marriage which as will be shown below is desirable. Saying no to gifts is also another possibility to avoid this dilemma and yet it seems this would threaten the very basis of relationships which function through generalised exchange and reciprocity. Besides, as will be shown below, gifts have other key uses in young women's lives so that saying no to the gift means saying no to the relationship which does not look like a viable option.

The Use of Gifts: Challenges of 'Emerging Femininity' Enhanced by Market-Based Products

Cash gifts are invested in modern toiletries in the form of facial creams and perfumed lotions imported from South Africa, Botswana or up north from Zambia. In the case of products from Zambia, some of them trace their origins from as far as West Africa.[14] Perfumed lotions double as skin care products and perfume to prevent body odour which was roundly said to be unpleasant, embarrassing and a turn-off for men. Facial lotions are usually vanishing creams which promise to remove blemishes, control oiliness and shininess and/or even out skin tone and texture. These attributes are much sought after. Some of the preferred facial creams are skin lighteners or bleaches which although banned are increasingly being smuggled into the country by cross-border traders. In FGDs I observed girls whose faces were much lighter than their necks and hands, suggesting the use of skin lighteners. Of course, such girls also had the much-coveted clear and smooth skin. The need for modern toiletries was indicated as one of the reasons why boys and men give money and girls and young women receive it. There is therefore considerable pressure placed on boys to deliver resources.[15]

Petroleum jelly, which is the cheapest form of skin care product on the market, unfortunately seems to create the opposite it leads to oiliness, encourages acne and blemishes thereof. Repondents complained that they could not use petroleum jelly referred to as 'vaseline' because of those undesirable effects. They prefer 'ponds'.[16] Petroleum jelly is said to be suitable for little girls. In spite of this apparent rejection, petroleum jelly remains the most affordable skin care products on the market. Shiminess and acne apparently turn-off potential male partners. They point to lack of sophistication. Girls who cannot afford commercially available products can use traditional alternatives such as lightly applying red ochre locally called 'isibhuda'[17] while the face is still moist after washing. It gives a 'matte' look similar to using modern foundation or face powder. In addition, girls said that the use of facial creams is also because of peer pressure. When other girls have 'beautiful faces', one feels out of place if one's face looks shiny or blemished.

Traditional beauty products are seen as unsophisticated, laborious to make and store. They are scentless or lack modern chemical smells. In one FGD, girls discussed traditional skin care products like mfuma.[18] They complained that mfuma smells badly. Some claimed it 'attracts flies' on account of the sour milk smell, others complained that 'it is for old women' or is 'old fashioned'. In FGDs with parents, women confirmed that most teenagers do not like mfuma although they also admitted that they too no longer make it. It is too much effort while others said they do not have access to adequate milk to make it. Most parents and guardians consider commercially available toiletries extra expenses and luxuries in a context where bread and butter issues are more pressing.

Some young women claimed not to use anything on their faces in order to minimise skin reactions. Others claimed to use the desired facial creams on and off depending on the availability of money. Some share creams with less fortunate girls. The latter use these creams on days and occasions when one must look different or beautiful to make an impression. Trips to the shops during weekends, errands during which one is likely to meet peers, or holidays when male migrants are back from Botswana and South Africa, were mentioned as occasions when one looks one's best. There were animated debates about how to have a 'beautiful skin' at low cost, including which soaps to use and not to use. However with or without money it was pointed out that women have look beautiful, 'ukuceca', using whatever one has and that many young women try by all means to look their best.

Money is also needed for underwear; 'beautiful underwear'. Girls indicated that older female siblings, where available, provided underwear as did mothers. However, there were complaints that mothers, especially, buy utilitarian panties, nothing 'lacy', in see-through synthetic materials. Examples were given of cheap underwear one finds at flea markets in the provincial capital which might be hard-wearing but far from 'beautiful'. The girls appreciated that this is the best their mothers could do. Respondents with older sisters in wage work could expect other types of underwear. The best choice was always where one chose the underwear onself but this implies having one's own income. Cash gifts from male partners came in handy in this instance. There were complaints that bras are particularly expensive and yet once one develops breasts 'clothes do not fit well without a bra'. The participant who made this contribution illustrated with her hands the movement of the breasts, to giggles of those present. The girls also complained that when one has a big bust it attracts attention if not well strapped up in a bra. In addition, girls need half-slips to wear with see-through clothes as part of female decency and propriety. However, girls noted that one cannot communicate such issues with fathers because of the norms of social distance between parents and children of the opposite sex. On the other hand, mothers might not have enough income to meet such needs. Some participants who are single mothers noted that once you have a child out of wedlock parents tend to say 'zibonele' — literally 'stand on you own feet' or 'be independent' — which implores youths to take care of themselves even when without tangible means of earning income. The same was observed in Tanzania by Kutapa (1998). This is because of a patrilineal ethos in which girls marry out and are expected to join their husband's families where all their material needs are met. Failure to get married forced young women to raise children in their families of birth often under conditions of resources austerity in which personal needs are not well met. This is part of the reason why some young women with children are pushed into transactional sex or sex for gifts as a means of meeting personal needs even when they get a roof and food from their parents. Parents feel that after a certain age they cannot continue to provide personal needs such as toiletries, sanitary ware and underwear, especially for daughters with children out of wedlock.

As mentioned above, 'growing up' for women signals the onset of menstruation which is an added expense because sanitary ware is now only really available through the market. There is very little known about traditional sanitary ware since women of different generations do not seem able to discuss these issues.[19] There is reason to think that many families simply do not factor this aspect in the family budget. Among poor families this is not possible on account of resource austerity. Girls learn not to make demands due to poverty but nature does not care much for poverty and menstruation becomes a monthly nightmare to be managed somehow. In a Zimbabwe Women's Resource Centre and Network (ZWRCN) study done several years ago, some girls from poor urban families missed school to stay at home until their period was over because they could not bear the thought of being at school without adequate sanitary ware. Girls in this study indicated that mothers and female siblings do buy sanitary ware when and if they have enough money. However, for economic reasons, female kin often decide the quantity of sanitaryware nevermind what the user's levels of comfort and needs might be. Otherwise, the girls are left to their own devices. Respondents indicated that cash gifts from boyfriends also go towards buying sanitaryware.

Another important item is soap. Toiletries and beauty routines mentioned above imply a certain amount of washing and cleansing of self and clothing. Generally, soap ('isepa') is considered a basic commodity. Many families strive to get it. Most would consider themselves deprived if they could not afford it. Basic soap comes in the form of a bar of up to 35 centimetres of multipurpose soap. Such bars tend to have a bland chemical smell. Although usable and effective as far as hygiene is concerned, these soaps are not liked. Girls talked about the need to buy their own soaps, usually perfumed bath soaps for personal use.

Gifts and their Implications for 'Safe Sex'

Gifts are equated with a steady relationship based on mutual trust. Gifts and sex seem to go together — which precludes the A (abstinence) of prevention messages. Abstinence was described as 'impossible' in the long term for any human being. Participants also indicated that there are women who are nymphomaniacs ('abelesagweba'). Such women are said to want to have sex daily and hence some of them are involved in commercial sex work. However, it was explained that avoiding sex (perceived as penetrative penile-vaginal sex) means finding alternative ways of managing sexual urges or feelings locally called 'imizwa'. Asked what these might be, there were no conclusions: whatever 'alternatives' that were suggested such as touching and kissing were seen as somehow incomplete. In some groups they were simply laughed off. Within relationships being faithful and 'sticking to one partner' with whom one can have sex is assumed to be acceptable. In most groups participants gave the impression that this was the meaning of the B (being faithful) and sticking to one partner. Youths said, in so many words, 'ukuba lomngane oyedwa othembikileyo' (that is, having one trustworthy partner). In reality female youths have several 'one partners' in a series and sometimes concurrently to maximize gifts. The gifts also tend to compromise the possibility of the use of condoms — the C of message. There were complaints too about some men not wanting to use condoms because 'condoms are dirty' ('ayidoti'). Asked to explain how this is so, respondents pointed to problems with the disposal of condoms, given that most youths have sex in unconventional places such as in the forests during the day or at night, in the fields or on streambeds which do not have appropirate facilities to dispose of condoms.[20] Some parents complained of used condoms strewn on streambeds. The condoms are eventually washed into dams. This contaminates the water with a high risk of livestock swallowing condoms. In two FGDs (one for girls and another for boys) there were questions about the female condom, what it looks like and where it is found. In the FGD with boys, one participant expressed anxiety about the danger of witchcraft if the condom is widely used. He raised this issue after asking for an explanation of how the condom works. He was concerned about a contraceptive which women control and one in which men literally leave their semen.[21]

In as much as gifts are a sign of commitment, condoms are thought to undermine it as they are associated with infidelity, transient relations and promiscuity. Condoms therefore threaten relationships, especially the possibility of marriage. Girls said that if a man spends a lot of money on a girl it seems 'unfair' or 'impossible' (stated as '... ungeke...', which means '...you cannot...') to demand condom use. It seems that to demand condom use under these circumstances points to a lack of gratitude. Girls pointed out that commitment itself is transitory as a male partner might find another 'better' female partner and shift his attention. They also noted that gifts as a sign of commitments are promissory but say nothing about men's readiness for long-term commitment and how men will respond to pregnancies which readily occur when sex is not condomised. Some girls said that having sex on men's terms is necessary to 'keep the relationship going' in anticipation of marriage. It also says that the woman is obedient and is herself marriageable (see Mate forthcoming on male youth masculinities and sexualities). Some also indicated that the promise of marriage is a ploy to get girls to agree to unsafe sex, but men and boys lose

94

interest once there is a pregnancy, leaving girls to face the music on their own (see also Kutapa 1998). Often notions of reciprocity are then construed as looseness in which the girls are blamed for failure to control themselves and their sexual urges, or stupidity and gullibility for failing to see through men's flimsy marriage promises.

The foregoing already presupposes that the need for safe sex is understood but its practice hinges on local notions of propriety and fairness. In keeping with discourses of awareness, respondents in this study are well aware of HIV and AIDS and how it is prevented. They could describe opportunistic symptoms associated with the latter stages of HIV infection. Many are aware that having multiple partners (concurrently) increases the possibility of being infected with HIV if one does not use condoms. On the other hand, 'sticking to one partner' was seen as a way of preventing HIV and AIDS. However when asked to think of multiple partners in a series, participants in different FGDs were doubtful or hesitant. They said that breaking up with one partner and moving on to another is normal and inevitable as one searches for the ideal life partner. They were keen to show that HIV and AIDS afflict those of 'loose morals' or those who are 'not well behaved', ('nxa ungaziphathi'), which when understood in the local language is a broad term referring to 'lack of propriety', being ill-mannered broadly defined. It was explained that impropriety such as paid sex leads to HIV infection. Women who engaged in paid sex were described as 'lazy' ('amavila'), or 'love money too much', and that is why they sell sex. However when asked to explain why 'local female youths' exchange for sex for cash to buy toiletries, lunch and sanitary ware, the debate took different paths. Some blamed poverty for pushing women to such levels of desperation while others still maintained the need for 'restraint' even in the face of desperation, because these early beginnings might lead to full-time commercial sex work. Adults on the other hand say that girls 'love sweet things' (stated as 'bathanda ezimnandi') such as sweets, fizzy drinks, biscuits and potato crisps. However that phrase also means 'nice' or 'delicious food'.

Compared to male participants, female respondents were less conversant with STIs. Focus group participants claimed that 'shyness' (inhloni), 'stupidity' ('ubuthutha') makes women unable to tell when partners are infected women with STIs. Some girls did mention smelly discharges and sores as some symptoms. Others said it is difficult to look at a man's genitals before sex. This was said amidst a lot of laughter and uncomfortable giggles. In Ward 12, 'failure to look' was explained as 'shyness'; this led to a debate about shyness, in which one participant suggested that those who are shy should not have sex in the first place. Some girls said the problem is that women 'pretend to be decent', or more specifically 'to make oneself decent' (bayazichumisa) so that they do not ask their partners to use condoms even when they are aware that the men are promiscuous or have signs of STIs. In other words, even shyness is a strategy which is deployed to give the impression of decency and naiveté. Thus even if girls knew signs of STIs, they have no way of seeing them in the dark. In other instances religious teaching prohibit the use of condoms. In both research sites, there is a sizable population of adherents of a religious sect which prohibits the use of hospitals and products associated with the including all forms of western medicine and contraceptives.

Marriage: the Ultimate Goal of Dating

All female participants, including those in difficult or failed marriages, roundly expressed aspirations for (re)marriage. They said that marriage is an ideal institution for women as it allows them to have their own homes or homesteads ('umuzi'), children, their own fields and to be 'complete', 'proper', and even 'respectable' women ('umfazi opheleleyo'). Marriage also prevents one from being promiscuous or being lured into commercial sex work. In so many ways marriage also offers girls a legitimate avenue to independence and social status (Kutapa 1998). Respondents said that men respect married women whereas single women have to contend with male attention tempting the women to get into casual sexual relationships. Some respondents countered that even married women are tempted to have casual sexual relations to revenge their husbands' promiscuity. FGD participants agree that for married women the penalty for extramarital affairs is heady, including divorce, labeling and lack of sympathy from the public. However, as already indicated, the way they go about it is such that it minimizes the achievement of this goal. An unskilled woman may have several boyfriends and fall pregnant along the way, leaving her bereft of any support. Older persons expressed indignation about such girls, saying they would not want such a daughter-in-law, nor would they like their own daughters to behave in this manner. They also claimed that in fact because of entrepreneurial dating once a girl falls pregnant, it is a matter of time before 'illness' (implying HIV and AIDS) comes. One participant expressed the sequence of events as '... ungabona isisu umkhuhlane ususondele' (that is, 'once there is a pregnancy, then illness is about to strike as well'). It suggests that in the process of falling pregnant (a by-product of trying to secure a husband) some girls get infected. Once the women is sick, she becomes a burden on her parents. After she dies the same parents bear the costs of the funeral and the expense of caring for children of the deceased. As a result, older persons think that marriage is ideal provided it is contracted 'the proper way' and is not preceded by premarital sex. Although female respondents in this study agree, they have not been able to confront their parents on the pressures they face so that some middle ground can be found in order to reduce risk. They too seek to achieve the goal of marriage, but are derailed by hazards inherent in the process.

Discussion

The foregoing illustrates the contradictions of the transformation of sexuality in a context where the lineage retains a vested interest in the individual but has no effective means of controlling behaviour (see Ahlberg 1994: 233; Foucault 1978). This change is supposedly a product of modernisation. It is clear that parental concerns and aspirations speak more of ideals of the past which are no longer supported by today's living arrangements and pressures. When youths have personal needs for 'modern' toiletries and sanitary ware and parental resources fall short, there is an issue to be resourced. Besides parents say 'zibonele' (fend for yourself) although the youths have no skills to sell and there are no visible employment opportunities. Calls for youths to find for themselves' push youths to creativing and resourcefulness which includes transactional sex. This change can be described as a kind of false modernity in which consumption of the worldly goods, individual rights and privacy are key. In this context modernity is about one's ability to consume goods that are 'modern', 'new', 'foreign', as a way of embracing traits that are 'with the world' (Friedman 1996). For women specific forms of packaging oneself and presenting the body for the 'male gaze' (Fuglesang 1994). As a consequence, those girls that are still using 'isibhuda' and 'mfuma' can be laughed off as old fashioned and unsophisticated, as are girls who cannot manage their acne.

In rural areas such as in this research site, 'privacy' is conflated with silence, inaction, indifference and ignorance, which all feed off each other and create a situation where more youths remain vulnerable to HIV and AIDS. Older people feel that they can no longer reprimand other people's children because of newfound notions of privacy, and because of the breakdown of the essence of the extended family and kinship. Uncles and aunts no longer have the ability, opportunity and maybe the interest to talk to their nieces and nephews. Within families parents are yet to learn how to talk about issues that are deeply personal and intimate with children. Thus sexualities that we observe on the ground are decidedly new and evolving. The talk about people failing to change their behaviour because of tradition or culture is therefore erroneous. The problem is that of modernity at the periphery, where people do not have similar resources to those at 'the centre', although through the media and other channels they internalise 'modern' values and norms such as individuality, privacy, consumption and commensurate notions of beauty.

It is also clear that adolescence and teenage years are a time when girls want their emerging femininity and sexuality acknowledged and taken seriously (McRobbie 1991). They embrace it and seek to enhance it with or without parental guidance. In a context where parents have no resources, the needs of these youths in this endeavour are seen as a luxury. The youth devise other means of accessing these goods through sex. In the West, where perhaps people have better resources, teenagers and the early twenty age groups are powerful markets for clothes and toiletries because manufacturers take advantage of this experimentation, the quest for self discovery and re-invention. In the Third World people also try to create new images of self. But lacking resources, the struggle is multi-layered. One does not only struggle to remake oneself but also to obtain the necessary resources to remake oneself. In the FGDs during this study there were many participants who wore hats known as 'sportie', popularised by South African township hip hop (kwaito) artists. The hat has a narrow visor but is worn low so that the eyes are partially covered. This is fashion associated with South African gangsters (tsotsis). Boys and girls wore the hats and often I had to ask them to adjust the hats so I could see their faces. Some girls wore corduroy berets in bright colours (imported from South Africa and Botswana) which could have been borrowed from sisters and friends for the occasion. Fashion is therefore important in the youths' lives with or without the resources that it demands.

When it comes to sanitary ware, girls are told that menstruation is a deeply private matter. Even when male partners give cash gifts it is understood to be for the girlfriend's 'discretionary spending'. Because most of us have no idea what older generations used during menstruation, to talk of the ideal past seems out of place when sanitary ware is now commercialised, girls engage in sport and have to continue to maintain this secret, which when not well-managed ceases to be a secret. When the councillor of Ward 17 asked for feedback on what our preliminary findings were, he was surprised to hear of sanitary ware and toiletries as an issue. In a discussion with him in the presence of six or so other local males, there was general acknowledgement of the fact that fathers 'do not know about these things' because they are not formally informed and do factor them into their budget. Some men, though, said it is not true that fathers are not aware because some of them have teenage girlfriends that they give money for discretionary spending while denying their daughters the same facilities. Some men felt that today's youths are 'out of control' ('ungeke ubakwanise'), and that they do not fear[22] sex or seeing the naked body of a person of the opposite sex as older generations had. This was blamed on biology as a subject in the school curriculum which demystifies the human body and reproduction process. Indications are that youths in the study are sexually experienced. It is a situation that makes adults unhappy and anxious. Among the youths, the fact that discussions were laced with laughter and giggles whose meanings one cannot convey on paper, points to the fact that issues under discussion are common to all, but are embarrassing to come to terms with. This discomfort might be a result of the dissonance between prevailing HIV and AIDS prevention discourses which privilege abstinence among youths and the reality of the needs and pressures with which these youths have to deal. Abstinence is still defined as 'no sex before marriage' (Marindo et al., 2003), yet in the past there was 'non-penetrative' sex or thigh sex which allowed youths to manage sexual urges (imizwa). This also trained them in sexual restraint (Alhberg 1994; see also Heald 1995). This 'no sex' rule which is connected to the modernising effects of Christian morality, is, as youths themselves admit, 'not feasible' or 'not sustainable' over a long time. Furthermore, these youths live in a social context where marriage and parenthood are expected of them. For many, premarital pregnancy is the best way to expedite marriage.

Although girls are told to avoid intimate contact with boys and men there is the reality that sex is seen as a rite of passage into adulthood (Eaton et al., 2002). Sex is equated with nature and normal interactions between consenting 'grown up' males and females in heterosexual relations (Sikwibele et al., 2000). In local parlance, sex is referred to as 'ukudla kwabadala', that is, 'elders' food'.[23] As such sex is also something that one does to show that one is old enough. Still, sexually active youth are described as youths who 'know too much', or 'have lost their innocence', and their sexual behaviour is seen as inappropriate. It is locally described as 'ukuganga' or 'ukuxwala', which means being 'deviant', 'wild', 'out of control' and/or 'wayward'. Youths see it as inevitable, arguing that no parents in their right mind would encourage children to have sex. So parental lectures are also accepted as 'normal' parental duties while the youths have to cope with personal pressures which remain unacknowledged by the parents.

Whatever the merits and demerits of youth sexuality, vulnerability to HIV infection is a real concern. This vulnerability has to be understood within this context of poverty (even relative poverty), new notions of beauty, and consumption patterns which pressure girls to receive presents from males but then compromise their ability to demand the use of condoms lest this negates their show of gratitude (see also Schoepf 1995 for DRC ; Nyanzi et al, 2000 for Uganda). On the other hand, parents who in keeping with local norms cannot look for partners for their daughters, aspire for sons-in-law with means. So young women are strategic in dating and target local professionals and enterprising persons capable of earning money through other means. Such dating frees parents of parental obligations to provide even though they pay dearly later when their daughters are sick. Men understand these economic expectations and make a point of displaying their relative wealth. Kutapa (1998) reports that the situation is the same in Dar es Salaam, Tanzania. In a rural setting such as the study site, buying fizzy and alcoholic drinks at local shops and drinking clear beer when others are drinking traditional opaque brews is a sign of status and the availability of disposable income. Thus in the research site, reports by male respondents indicate that during the holidays when migrants working in South Africa and Botswana return home, the competition for girls stiffens. The migrants have more disposable income and can buy drinks, sweets and biscuits, outdoing local competition.

Exchange of gifts clearly puts girls in a bind where they are obliged to reciprocate. Failure to reciprocate is seen as immoral, selfish and justifies male violence (see also Varga 1997 for KwaZulu-Natal, South Africa). As observed by Dover (2002), 'propriety' of behaviour is often expressed in terms of appropriateness of gender roles. In other words, women who get gifts and are not keen on reciprocity are also saying that they are not marriageable since they do not maintain their side of the bargain. They take advantage of men and therefore send the wrong message to likely suitors. Thus although premarital sex is seen by many parents as inappropriate, it resonates well with existing marriage models which ideally revolve around the economically empowered male attached to an economically disempowered female raising children together. Their needs feed off each other, creating mutuality. Men usually want the 'comforts of home' (sex, domestic work done for them) while women want money to care for the children by meeting men's needs.

Due to the fact that male-female sexual relations are characterised by wit, shrewdness, deceit and lies, (Varga 1997; Eaton et al., 2003; Nnko and Pool 1997; Chikovore et.al, 2002; Mate 2005), the promise of marriage is used to get females to agree to sex on unfavourable terms. When a pregnancy occurs the women are left in the lurch. Some women, too, lie and double-cross to maximize returns, but still want marriage to ensure a good social standing in adult life. Thus, although premarital pregnancy is risky in that it does not guarantee that one gets married, it remains the commonest way of initiating marriage (see Chikovore et al., 2002). A pregnancy usually leads to an elopement after which marriage negotiations are initiated.[24] Once a young woman is pregnant, parents have no choice but to accept a marriage offer because otherwise children born out of wedlock to single women increase the economic burden on the woman's family. A marriage offer is important to resolve the tension otherwise created by pregnancy out of wedlock. Besides, families fear that unmarried daugthers with children out of wedlock with fetch lower bride price in subsequent marriages because they are seen as 'spoiled' or 'damaged'. In addition, most men do not like the economic burden of looking after 'other men's children' ; so if the woman succeeds in getting married to another man, she is likely leave children from previous relationships with her parents. It remains a paradox that young women risk unplanned pregnancies in the hope of marriage which is not guaranteed. On the other hand, use of contraceptives increases the likelihood of being seen as loose and denies one the means by which to expedite marriage. Thus risking marriage (through unplanned pregnancies) also increases the risk of contracting HIV. This is a tight moral rope for young women to walk.

The foregoing need not portray youths as passive victims of poverty and changing culture per se. Sikwibele et al., (2000) noted in Northern Zambia that young women realise that economic pressures increase their dependence on men and compromise their health as they risk infection with HIV. 'Intellectual empowerment' (Baylies and Bujra 2000) does not seem to lead to decisions that minimize risks. Parents too have enough of this 'intellectual empowerment' to know that pregnancies in this generalised epidemic seem to predate illness. But like their daughters, they seem unable to do anything about the situation. In this study, girls debated men well enough to show that they are aware that cheating is par for the course, they realise that 'commitment' is transitory, and that marriage may be promised but will not materialise. Some girls engage in multiple partner sex in order to maximize cash returns and to hedge against dead-end relationships that do not lead to marriage. However due to the tyranny of physiology, it is women who carry the burden of pregnancy and display the evidence of 'impropriety'. Confusion about who the father of the child is reduces chances of marriage. After the child is born, the father is not keen to assist in raising a child and so the girls are pushed more and more towards transactional sex as a livelihood strategy (Hunter 2002). However, none of the girls referred to this behaviour overtly as commercial sex work. They all decried their consumerist needs — for confectionery, toiletries and underwear — which parents and guardians think are luxurious extras, but which they themselves see as basics. In the process, the practice of safe sex is sabotaged.

Notwithstanding the amount of work done by HIV and AIDS prevention programmes, myths about condoms still abound. There is a belief that condoms have 'germs' because of local experiments performed with condoms (Caldwell 2000). Sikwibele et al., (2000) also report that in Northern Zambia youths claim that condoms apparently have pores which allow viral matter to flow into the blood. Mate (2002) also reports that in parts of Zimbabwe people distrust free condoms and claim that they are laced with the HIV virus. In the FGDs, these myths took on a new meaning when some participants asked exactly how the condom prevents pregnancy and HIV infection. At issue here are the mechanics of condoms as a barrier method. To the best of my knowledge no one explains these things when teaching about condoms: what is it about a condom that prevents infection? Sometimes when people do not understand how something works, the nitty-gritty of its mechanics, they cannot use it. Another problem is condom disposal given prevalent views and attitudes towards secretions from human genitalia. Most rural youth have sex in secluded outdoor locations such as woods en route to or from school, on streambeds or in the fields or while running errands for their parents. This means that one must either carry the used condom home or to a pit latrine. Alternatively one leaves it there in the forest, thereby exposing one's intimate secretions. Indeed used condoms were reported in the woods and streambeds with some adults worrying that they are a menace to their livestock, especially goats and cows.

Condom use is also made impossible by very real inhibitions such as their expensive nature. At the time of doing fieldwork, condoms cost Z$50,000 for a pack of three in the study area, although the same pack cost Z$10,000 in major towns. Given poverty and other demands on people's income, condoms are likely to be ignored. Although there are free condoms at clinics, with distances of between 20 to 30 kilometres (Langhuag et al. 2003) to the nearest health centre, it is highly unlikely that youths will take the trouble to obtain the condoms. How would one explain the reason for the journey to one's parents or guardians? There are also observations that rural clinics in Africa as a whole are public spaces where the physical set-up does not allow for privacy (Bledsoe and Cohen 1993; Langhaug et al., 2003). In Zimbabwe clinics make a habit of putting condoms in open spaces at the reception so that whoever picks them up does so publicly. For school-going youths, going to the clinic requires authorisation from school and clinics are known either to report to schools what their students' complaints are or schools demand these records as part of monitoring children in their care. Since many adults consider that youths are not supposed to engage in sex unless married, youth access to condoms through such public facilities is fraught with problems (Betts et al., 2000; Meekers and Molathlegi 2001). Although there are Village Community Workers (VCWs) who among other things also distribute condoms, they are local villagers who apparently are judgmental of youths who want them. The VCWs are afterall older persons who are likely to talk about the 'waywardness' of so-and-so's child. Youth felt that the likelihood of the VCWs reporting them to their parents or the news reaching their parents through the village grapevine was very high.

Conclusion

By referring to 'perfumed lotions, biscuits and condoms', this paper has tried to show that the consumption needs and lifestyles of youths negate condom use or safe sex. The gifts which allow them access to lotions and biscuits oblige them to engage in unsafe sex. Thus the increased salience of transactional sex and the accompanying spread of HIV can easily lead to people thinking that 'African sexualities' are undisciplined, when in reality this change is in tandem with global trends of individuality, consumerism and the overall logic of the market (Hunter 2002; Ugarteche 2000). As noted above, the transactional sex observed in this study is bound up with notions of femininity, poverty and the need to get ahead in an environment where nothing else seems viable. Everywhere female youths have the 'intellectual empowerment' (Baylies and Bujra 2000) to understand issues about HIV and AIDS and male-female relations, but they lack viable alternatives for achieving their personal aspirations through means that are less risky. Thus HIV and AIDS prevention among the youth is not as easy as ABC. The reality is more complex. It is not enough to focus on sexual acts and omit the socio-cultural and economic contexts. Otherwise well intentioned HIV and AIDS strategies miss their targets.

Notes

1. ABCDEFG = Abstain, Be faithful to an uninfected partner, Correct and consistent use of Condoms, Delay early sex, Early treatment of sexually transmitted infections, Free and frank discussion, Get real and know your HIV status. (Corridors of Hope/USAID poster displayed in health facilities in Zimbabwe from 2004).
2. For the purposes of this study, youths are people aged between 15 and 24 years of age in keeping with the UN definition.
3. There are some chieftaincies that have tried to have virginity tests for girls and a certification process of sorts. This has accentuated the girls' vulnerability to men who believe that sex with a virgin has medicinal values or brings a man luck.
4. The critique of 'ladette culture' in the UK is a case in point here. 'Ladettes' are hedonistic young women who behave like 'the lads' through excessive alcohol consumption, drug use and multiple partner sex that supposedly belie the 'freedoms', 'choices', 'opportunities' and increased income which today's

women enjoy. This development has left older generations of feminists asking whether indeed this is a manifestation of the feminist vision of gender equality they imagined.

5. A ward is an administrative unit comprising of between six and eight villages and is represented by an elected official called a councillor. The councillor represents the villages at the Rural District Council (RDC) which is the local authority in a rural area.

6. Poor communication of dates and venues led to clashes in two sites in Ward 12, making us miss one of the meetings.

7. In FGDs with adults, fathers complained that often they are not formally told that their daughters 'are grown up' or 'have become women' and only know that this is the case when the girl becomes pregnant. They complained that this is because traditional kinship ties have waned so that their sisters no longer play the key roles expected of them within the lineage.

8. Sanitary ware for women is generally very expensive in Zimbabwe as most products are imported. Even the most basic product like cotton wool are not affordable for many women in households already reeling under the pressure of poverty. Investing in sanitary ware is an extra expense which most households consider a luxury rather than an essential.

9. The 'Mai Chisamba Show' on whether or not neighbours and friends should report real or suspected misdemeanours of friends and relatives' spouses or children.

10. Male respondents also indicated that they feel pressured to give gifts as a way of staking a claim to a girl, showing responsibility and obliging girls to acquiesce to sex.

11. They are usually returned when a relationship ends.

12. In rural areas, schoolchildren take packed lunches of watermelons when in season, boiled sweet potatoes, dry maize boiled together with dry pulses among others. During school functions like sports days there are usually a lot of other goodies on sale such as fizzy drinks, biscuits, sweets etc.

13. A cheap sweetened and artificially coloured drink frozen in a tubular plastic. It is like an ice-lolly. Shop owners with freezers sell them to local people to quell the heat. They are a favourite of many children.

14. They reach Zimbabwe through complex networks of cross-border trade of Nigerians, Congolese, Zambian and Zimbabwean traders.

15. FGDs with male youths indicate that they feel pressured to give cash gifts to girlfriends to make them 'look beautiful'.

16. Although this is a brand name of an international range of beauty products, it is used locally to refer to a variety of facial preparations.

17. Also used by women to decorate mud huts. It is mixed with water to apply to walls.

18. This is made from evaporated dairy cream leaving only a fatty residue which is applied on the skin, especially in winter. It does prevent chafing, flaking of the skin associated with cold weather. Because mfuma is a by-product in the making of sour milk, it tends to have a distinct sour milk-like smell. My recollections of using it as a child (in my pre-teens) are not that pleasant. I preferred the bland modern petroleum jelly to mfuma.

19. Also, menstruation is considered a deeply private matter so that when a local women's NGO lobbied the government to reduce tariffs on sanitary ware, some women thought the NGO had crossed boundaries of propriety by discussing such aspects of women's lives publicly in parliament.

20. Implied here are fears of witchcraft, especially in connection with the disposal of intimate body fluids such as semen. Leaving a used condom in the forest means leaving one's body fluids lying around in a rubber pouch! It makes people feel very vulnerable. The alternative would be to carry the used condom all the way home and throw it in a pit latrine, assuming there is one. However, this also means one has to have appropriate packaging for the used condom.

21. Women apparently can use semen to make potent love portions; the kind that ensure that the man stays faithful or shuns other women.

22. The word fear is used rather literally to equate to the vernacular phrase 'kabayesabi'. However, in the context of their discussion it can be understood to describe 'eagerness that it imbued with recklessness'.

23. In the past, this included local delicacies such as types of game meat which children were not allowed to eat. Often there were myths about what would happen to children who broke the bounds of propriety with regard to this food. Over the years, people have learnt that these are empty myths. The taboos no longer hold.

24. Although not included in this study, most poor young men prefer this type of marriage initiation because if they use other means, namely to ask for a girl's hand in marriage when she is not pregnant, parents may well refuse on account of the man's poverty or low status.

References

Ahlberg, B. M., 1994, 'Is there a Distinct African Sexuality?: A Critical Response to Caldwell', *Africa*, vol. 64, no. 2, pp. 220-242.

Barnett, T., and Whiteside, A., 2002, *AIDS in the Twenty First Century: Disease and Globalization*, London, Palgrave.

Baylies, C., et al., 1999, 'Rebels at Risk: Young Women and the Shadow of AIDS in Africa', in C. Becker et al., eds., *Experiencing and Understanding AIDS in Africa*, pp. 321-341, Dakar: CODESRIA.

Baylies, C., and Bujra. J., 2000, 'The Struggle Continues', in Baylies, C. and Bujra. J., eds., AIDS, *Sexuality and Gender in Africa: Collective Strategies and Struggles in Tanzania and Zambia*, London, Routledge.

Betts, S. C., et al., 2003, 'Zimbabwean Adolescents' Condom Use: what Makes the Difference? Implications for Intervention', *Journal of Adolescent Health*, vol. 33, pp. 165-171.

Bledsoe, C., and Cohen, B., 1993, *Social Dynamics of Adolescent Fertility in Sub-Saharan Africa*, Washington DC, National Academy Press.

Bond, V., 1997, '«Between a Rock and Hard Place»: Applied Anthropology and AIDS Research on a Commercial farm in Zambia', *Health Transitions Review*, supplement 3 to vol. 7.

Caldwell, J. C., 2000, 'Rethinking the African AIDS Epidemic', *Population and Development Review*, vol. 26, no. 1, pp. 117-135.

Chikovore, J., et al., 2002a, 'In their Own Words: Young People's Experiences, Concerns and Dilemmas in Sexual and Reproductive Health in a Prohibitive and Silent Context in Zimbabwe'.

Chikovore, J., et al., 2002b, 'Denial and Violence: Paradoxes in Men's Perspectives to Premarital sex and Pregnancy in Rural Zimbabwe'.

Crewe, M., 2004, Presentation at the Review Conference for the Global Youth Fellowship 2003/4, University of Pretoria, South Africa.

Dilger, H., 2001, 'AIDS in Africa: Broadening the Perspectives on Research and Policy-Making', *Afrika Spectrum*, vol. 36, no. 1, pp. 5-16.

Dover, P., 2002, 'Morality and Misfortune: Discourses Around ill Health in a Zambian Village', *SIDA Studies*, no. 7, pp. 160-169.

Dowsett, G. W., et al., 1998, 'Changing Gender Relations Among Young People: the Global Challenge for HIV/AIDS Prevention', *Critical Public Health*, vol. 8, pp. 291-309.

Friedman, J., 1996, 'Being in the World: Globalization and Localization', in Featherstone, M., ed., *Global Culture*, London, Sage Publications.

Foucault, M., 1978, *The History of Sexuality*, New York, Random House.

Fuglesang, M., 1994, *Veils and Videos: Female Youth Culture on the Kenyan Coast*, Stockholm.

Goldthorpe, J. E., 1983, *The Sociology of the Third World: Disparity and Development*, Cambridge, Cambridge University Press.

Government of Zimbabwe (GoZ), 1999, *National HIV/AIDS Strategic Framework*, Harare, Government Printers.

Heald, S., 1995, 'The Power of Sex: Some Reflections on the Caldwells "African Sexuality" Thesis' in *Africa*, vol. 65, no.4, pp.489-505.

Hunter, M., 2002, 'The Materiality of Everyday Sex: Thinking Beyond "Prostitution" in *African Studies*, vol. 61, number 2, pp.99-120.

Holton, R. J., 1998, *Globalization and the Nation-state*, London, Macmillan.

IDS-UNDP, 2003, *The Zimbabwe Human Development Report – Redirecting our responses to HIV and AIDS*, Harare, IDS.

Jewkes, R. K., et al., 2003, 'Gender inequalities, Intimate Partner Violence and HIV Preventive Practice: Findings of a South African Cross Sectional Study', *Social Science and Medicine* vol. 56, no. 1, pp. 125-134.

Kaler, A., 2003, '"My Girlfriends could Fill a Yanu-yanu Bus": Rural Malawian Men's claims about their Own Serostatus', *Demographic Research*, 19 September, available at www.DemographicResearch Marx-Planck-Gesellschaft

Kutapa, R., 1998, 'Teenage Mothers in their Second Pregnancies', in Rwebangira, M. K., and Liljeström, R., eds., *'Haraka, Haraka... Look Before You Leap: Youths at the Crossroad of Custom and Modernity'*, Uppsala, SIAS.

Kitzinger, J., 1994, 'Focus Groups: Method or Madness', in Boulton, Mary, ed., *Challenge and Innovation: Methodological Advances in Social Research on HIV/AIDS*, London, Taylor and Francis.

Langhaug, L. F., et al., 2003, 'Improving Young People's Access to Reproductive Healthcare in Rural Zimbabwe', *AIDS Care*, vol. 15, no. 2, pp. 147-157.

Marindo, R., et al., 2003, 'Condom use and Abstinence among Unmarried Young People in Zimbabwe: Which Strategy and Whose Agenda?', A Population Council Working paper number 170, available at www.popcouncil.org/pdfs/wp/170.pdf (accessed November 2004)

Mate, R., 2002, Individuals, Households/Families and Communities' Perceptions of and Responses to HIV/AIDS Infection, its Prevention and its Effects: Lessons for a more Grounded Strategy? UNDP-Poverty Reduction Forum Research paper for the 2003, Zimbabwe Human Development Report.

Mate, R., 2005, 'Making Ends Meet at the Margins?: Grappling With Economic Crisis and Belonging in Beitbridge Town, Zimbabwe', Dakar, CODESRIA Discussion Paper Series.

McRobbie, A., 1991, *Feminism and Youth Culture*, London, Macmillan.

Meekers, D., Ahmed, G., and Molathlegi, M. T., 2001, 'Understanding Constraints to Adolescent Condom Procurement: the Case of Urban Botswana', *AIDS Care*, no. 3, pp. 297-302.

Nelson, N., 1987, '«Selling her Kiosk»: Kikuyu Notions of Sexuality and Sex for Sale in Mathare Valley, Kenya', in Caplan, P., ed., *The Cultural Construction of Sexuality*, London, Routledge.

Nnko, S., and Pool, R., 1997, 'Sexual Discourses in the Context of AIDS: Dominant Themes on Adolescent Sexuality Among Primary School Pupils in Magu district, Tanzania', *Health Transitions Review*, Supplement 3 to vol. 7.

Nyanzi, S., Pool, R., and Kinsman, J., 2000, 'The Negotiation of Sexual Relationships Among School Pupils in South Western Uganda', *AIDS Care*, vol. 13, no. 1, pp. 83-96.

Pollak, M., 1992, 'AIDS: a Problem for Sociological Research: Introduction', *Current Sociology*, vol. 40, no. 3, pp. 1-10.

Schoepf, B. G., 1995, 'Culture, Sex Research and AIDS Prevention in Africa', in H. ten Brummelhuis and G. Herdt, eds., *Culture and Sexual Risk: Anthropological Perspectives on AIDS*, Gordon and Breach Publishers.

Sikwibele, A., et al., 2000, 'AIDS in Kapulanga, Mongu: Poverty, Neglect and Gendered Patterns of Blame', in Baylies, C., and Bujra, J., eds., *AIDS, Sexuality and Gender in Africa: Collective Strategies and Struggles in Tanzania and Zambia*, London, Routledge.

Simbayi, L. C., et al., 2004, 'Behavioural Responses of South African Youth to the HIV/AIDS Epidemic: A Nationwide Survey', *AIDS Care*, vol. 16, no. 5, pp. 605-618.

Scorgie, F., 2002, 'Virginity Testing and the Politics of Sexual Responsibility: Implications for AIDS Interventions' in African Studies, vol. 61, no.1, pp.55-75.

Ugarteche, C., 2000, *The False Dilemma: Globalisation Opportunity or Threat?*, London, Zed Books.

Van Eeuwijk, B., and Mlanga, S., 1997, 'Competing Ideologies: Adolescence, Knowledge and Silences in Dar es Salaam', in Harcourt, W., ed., *Power, Reproduction and Gender: the Intergenerational Transfer of Knowledge*, London, Zed Books.

Varga, C., 1997, 'Sexual Decision Making and Negotiation in the Midst of AIDS: Youth in KwaZulu Natal, South Africa', *Health Transitions Review*, Supplement 3 to vol. 7, pp. 46-67.

Weiss, B., 1993, '"Buying her Grave": Money, Movement and AIDS in North-West of Tanzania', *Africa*, vol. 33, pp. 19-35.

Zinyama, L., 2000, 'Who, What, When and Why: Cross Border Movement from Zimbabwe to South Africa' in McDonald DA (eds.) On Borders: Perspectives on International Migration in Southern Africa, St Martins Press, pp. 71-85.

Socio-Culture et VIH-SIDA au Cameroun

Antoine Socpa

Le VIH/SIDA représente l'un des plus grands défis de santé et de développement qui comporte un impact sur les bases sociales, économiques et démographiques du développement. Cette étude repose sur le postulat selon lequel la propagation du VIH en Afrique serait liée au comportement sexuel qui est fortement influencé par les facteurs socioculturels. Depuis plusieurs années, les débats sur les infections sexuellement transmissibles (IST) en général et le virus de l'immunodéficience humaine (VIH), responsable du syndrome d'immunodéficience acquise (SIDA) en particulier, rentrent dans un vaste champ de recherche multidisciplinaire. Ainsi, les spécialistes des sciences biomédicales et les chercheurs en sciences sociales sont invités à travailler sur divers aspects relevant de la sexualité, de la fécondité et de la santé de la reproduction. Cette interdisciplinarité et même cette trans-disciplinarité a l'avantage de rechercher aussi loin que possible l'origine et les causes de la maladie, surtout en ce moment où, face à l'absence de vaccin et de traitement efficace contre la pandémie, toutes les stratégies jusque-là envisagées sur le plan institutionnel ne sont pas encore parvenues à maîtriser la propagation continuelle du VIH/SIDA dans le monde en général et dans les pays pauvres en particulier. Pour le cas du Cameroun par exemple, des statistiques recueillies font état d'une progression sans cesse de la pandémie, avec une séroprévalence qui va de l'ordre de 0.5 pour cent en 1985 à environ 12 pour cent en 2002 et 5.5 pour cent depuis 2005. Face à ce phénomène, certaines études menées tendent à démontrer que les pratiques culturelles ont un rôle significatif à jouer si l'on veut agir sur l'état de santé d'une population. Aussi, est-il intéressant de s'interroger ici sur le lien (qui existe ou peut exister) entre les pratiques sexuelles dictées par une culture donnée et la propagation du virus responsable du SIDA. En d'autres termes, quelle corrélation existe-t-il entre les schèmes socioculturels d'une collectivité, ses mœurs et la propagation continuelle du VIH/SIDA ? Dans quelle mesure le changement de comportement à l'égard de ces pratiques culturelles influencerait-il les différents aspects de la propagation, du traitement et de la prise en charge de la pandémie ?

Cette réflexion s'appuie sur la considération générale selon laquelle l'élément culturel, sans être le seul facteur déterminant de la situation sanitaire d'une collectivité donnée, influence de manière significative le comportement sexuel des individus dans le sens de la prévention du VIH/SIDA, du traitement ou de la prise en charge des personnes infectées et/ou affectées par la maladie.

À ce titre, il serait intéressant de partir des tendances théoriques culturaliste et diffusionniste qui ont été utilisées au départ pour combler le vide théorique observé, afin de faire ressortir par la suite les facteurs explicatifs de la propagation du VIH/SIDA sous l'impulsion des éléments à la fois socioculturels, économiques et institutionnels liés à la dynamique culturelle et à l'urbanisation. Les données utilisées dans cet article proviennent à la fois de la littérature et des sources primaires, notamment des observations et des enquêtes qualitatives dans les provinces du centre et du nord du Cameroun.

Le VIH/SIDA comme phénomène social global

L'étude des facteurs de propagation du VIH/SIDA ainsi que de ses mécanismes de transmission ont permis à différentes disciplines scientifiques, usant de techniques, méthodes et résultats qui leur sont propres, de contribuer à la compréhension du phénomène en comblant un vide théorique observé à l'origine de l'épidémie (Touré 1995:135). En effet, les spécialistes des sciences sociales et biomédicales ont jeté leur dévolu dans la recherche sur le sida au détriment des études sur les pathologies infectieuses (Rosenheim et Itoua-Ngaporo 1989). L'ampleur de ces réflexions a fait de cette épidémie la « maladie du Siècle » tant il est vrai que presque toutes les instances de la société ont été interpellées. Qu'il s'agisse des décideurs, chercheurs de toutes les disciplines scientifiques, que des personnes infectées ou affectées par le VIH/SIDA.

La tâche dévolue aux sciences sociales était à ce titre d'apporter des éléments scientifiques à même d'expliquer les facteurs socioculturels empêchant toute maîtrise de l'épidémie. Il s'agissait à ce titre de venir en appui aux sciences biomédicales pour rechercher sous une forme plus globale des éléments sur l'origine sociale et les causes de la propagation vertigineuse de la maladie.

Approche culturo-fonctionnaliste et propagation du VIH/SIDA

Plusieurs documents (Nebout 1994, Rosenheim et Itoua-Ngaporo 1989) et rapports d'organismes (OMS, ONUSIDA, CNLS, etc.) font état non seulement de la situation épidémiologique mondiale du fléau (fréquence de l'infection, agents pathogènes, population à risque, etc.), mais aussi présentent des informations sur la nature du virus du SIDA (sa signification, sa provenance, son mode de pénétration dans l'organisme, etc.), ses modes de transmission (par des rapports sexuels, par voie sanguine, par transmission de la mère à l'enfant, etc.), les mécanismes de prévention (prévention de la transmission par le sang, par transfusion, par des seringues ou des instruments mal stérilisés, conseils aux donneurs de sang, méthodes contraceptives, etc.).

À ce titre, l'OMS estimait qu'environ dix millions de personnes étaient infectées en 1996 par le VIH, avec le continent africain comme région du monde la plus touchée avec près de 9/10e des enfants malades du SIDA. Cinq ans après, ce chiffre est passé de dix à au moins quarante millions de personnes infectées. Les régions d'Afrique les plus touchées par l'épidémie sont les pays de l'Afrique centrale, l'Afrique de l'Est et l'Afrique de l'Ouest.

Les premiers cas de VIH/SIDA ont été diagnostiqués au Cameroun en 1985. À cette période, le nombre de cas déclarés était de 21 personnes. Très vite, ce chiffre a suivi une ascension fulgurante. Il est en effet passé à 604 individus en 1991 pour atteindre 1761 en 1994 et ensuite 3950 individus en 1997. Le taux de prévalence estimé à 0,5 pour cent en 1987 est passé à 7,2 pour cent en 1999, puis à 11 pour cent en 2000. En 2003, le taux officiel de séroprévalence national était estimé à 12 pour cent et à 5.5 pour cent en 2005. Lorsqu'on considère la situation selon les groupes d'âges, les données relatives à l'année 2000 montrent que 12 pour cent de la population âgée entre 15 et 24 ans était porteur du virus. Au niveau de la tranche d'âge située entre 25 et 34 ans, le taux d'infection était de l'ordre de 9 à 10 pour cent. Au-delà de 35 ans cependant ce taux est le plus bas avec 8 pour cent de personnes infectées. Ainsi, il apparaît que la tranche d'âge de 20-24 ans avec 12,20 pour cent de personnes infectées est la plus touchée par la pandémie, suivie de celle de 15-19 ans avec 11,50 pour cent. Viennent ensuite les tranches d'âges de 25-29 ans (10 pour cent), de 30-34 ans (9,20 pour cent) et enfin les plus de 35 ans avec 8,10 pour cent de personnes infectées. Par ailleurs les données par sexe font ressortir un taux de prévalence de 11,7 pour cent chez les femmes (pour la plupart âgées entre 25 et 29 ans), contre 7,2 pour cent chez les hommes. La conclusion qui se dégage est que les femmes sont la couche de population la plus vulnérable à l'infection au VIH/SIDA. En général, les jeunes, notamment les filles libres, les prostituées, les camionneurs, les migrants, les ouvriers, les forestiers, les hommes en tenue (militaires, gendarmes, policiers) constituent la couche la plus exposée. Par ailleurs, la contamination de la mère à l'enfant, en l'absence de toute intervention, serait à elle seule responsable de plus de 20 000 nouvelles infections par an, soit 50 à 69 cas par jour chez l'enfant (CNLS 2001).

Le VIH/SIDA : une épidémie africaine à l'origine ?

Des préjugés ethniques et raciaux ont été véhiculés pour justifier l'origine africaine du VIH/SIDA, après que l'éventualité d'une origine simiesque de l'épidémie ait été écartée. Pour de nombreux Africains, le VIH-SIDA est la maladie de « l'homme Blanc », il est le produit des multiples manipulations transgéniques dont seuls les chercheurs occidentaux ont le secret (Sabatier 1989). Ces débats sur l'origine et surtout la propagation du virus, ses modes de transmission s'appuient sur le fait que les premières personnes touchées à travers le monde se retrouvent dans la plupart des cas, parmi la couche des populations démunies des « tropiques » et des exclus de la prospérité socio-économique des pays industrialisés.

Depuis près d'une décennie, les pratiques culturelles sont considérées comme des facteurs pouvant permettre d'expliquer le passage du virus de l'animal, principalement du singe africain à l'homme (Touré 1995). Cette conception culturaliste de l'origine du VIH/SIDA a été renforcée par la tendance diffusionniste selon laquelle, la propagation du virus est liée essentiellement au phénomène migratoire, avec notamment le déplacement des populations des zones rurales avec les singes vers les centres urbains. De ce fait, le niveau de vie précaire et la promiscuité ambiante des populations agglutinées dans des bidonvilles ne pouvaient que favoriser des comportements à risque et une dissémination de la maladie (Clumeck 1989). Pour ces raisons, les premières conclusions anthropologiques attribuaient la propagation vertigineuse du virus aux pratiques et comportements sexuels des Africains qui les rendraient plus vulnérables à cette maladie. Selon V. Kimani (1989), la promiscuité sexuelle inhérente à la culture africaine permet d'avoir plusieurs partenaires sexuels conformément aux règles qui régissent les institutions sociales et les pratiques fondées par les systèmes de filiation et de succession, d'une part, et le système de croyance y référant, d'autre part. De plus, la propagation du VIH est attribuée aux rapports hétérosexuels favorisés par les systèmes matrimoniaux polygamiques, le lévirat pour le cas de certaines sociétés africaines de type matrilinéaire et les croyances fondées sur le culte des ancêtres (Caldwell 1993 cité par Touré 1995). Comment peut-il en être autrement quand on sait que les rapports hétérosexuels en Afrique sont responsables de 80 pour cent des modes de transmission de la maladie.

Au demeurant, le fait que les rapports sexuels ne soient pas le propre des Africains conduit à relativiser les conclusions des thèses culturaliste et diffusionniste (Touré 1995:136), et comme tel, ne permet pas leur généralisation. Ce qui fait du déterminisme culturel fondé sur les rapports hétérosexuels une simple exagération de la réalité tant il est vrai que les multiples changements dont fait face l'Afrique subsaharienne ont nécessairement entraîné des transformations au niveau des « manières de penser, de sentir et d'agir » de toutes les couches de la population. Cette dynamique sociale touche amplement les pratiques dites traditionnelles au point de modifier ou d'altérer leur mode de fonctionnement et, par ricochet, participer à la propagation du VIH/SIDA en Afrique.

Valeurs traditionnelles, comportements sexuels et facteurs de propagation du VIH/SIDA

Les communautés qui peuplent l'Afrique sub-saharienne disposent d'un système de croyances, des institutions sociales et religieuses qui résistent tant bien que mal aux mutations qui affectent notre société contemporaine. C'est dire que quelle que soit la forme d'extraversion que peut subir une culture, il n'en demeure pas moins vrai que tout groupe socioculturel, comme le souligne Andezian (1985) :

> à sa manière spécifique d'appréhender et d'expliquer les notions de santé qui dépend étroitement de sa représentation du monde, de la vie, de la mort, de son système de croyance, de ses valeurs, de son rapport à l'environnement, de son univers relationnel.

Ces schèmes culturels, surtout ceux qui sont étroitement liés aux comportements sexuels, ont évolué avec le temps et entraîné par le fait même des répercussions sur la perception du VIH/SIDA, la propagation de la maladie et le traitement des malades. La littérature sur la sexualité en Afrique montre que certaines mœurs sexuelles prédisposent les femmes à une grande vulnérabilité par rapport aux hommes.

Mœurs sexuelles et vulnérabilité des femmes

De nombreuses études ont démontré que d'une manière générale, la femme est plus exposée que l'homme face aux risques de contamination par le virus du SIDA en cas de rapport sexuel non protégé ; pour la simple raison que le sperme infectée par le virus reste plus ou moins longtemps dans le conduit vaginal. Ces mêmes études soulignent que les jeunes filles et femmes sont plus exposées que leurs aînées aux infections dans la mesure où les cellules protectrices sont moins nombreuses dans le vagin et que le col de l'utérus est plus fragile. Dans ces conditions, certaines pratiques traditionnelles telles que le mariage précoce, les rapports sexuels extraconjugaux, le legs des femmes, et plusieurs rituels sexuels sont susceptibles d'accroître la vulnérabilité de la femme notamment en ce qui concerne sa santé reproductive.

Les pratiques relatives aux formes de sexualité rituelle et thérapeutique reposent sur une double idéologie. Celles de la production et de la reproduction.

Production agricole et sexualité

Une étude menée par l'African Population Advisory Committee–Cameroun (2004) –APAC, montre que la pratique de la sexualité rituelle est fréquente dans les communautés Mafa, Toupouri et Mousgoum dès le début des campagnes agricoles et piscicoles. En effet, à ces périodes précises, les paysans se livrent à une sexualité désordonnée, voire à un libertinage des rapports sexuels en vue de « faire en sorte que les récoltes ou les moissons soient bonnes ». Le fait d'entretenir des rapports sexuels rituels est culturellement prescrit par une croyance selon laquelle ils donnent la vie tout comme la terre donne la vie aux plantes. Cette pratique normative est décrite ici par un informateur traditionaliste :

> Quand les premières pluies commencent, les relations sexuelles sont encore normales. Mais quand c'est déjà les semences si tu as un champ, tu dois d'abord avoir les relations avant d'aller semer. C'est bon quand la femme avec qui tu vas aller a déjà accouché ; là, la terre va produire beaucoup... pendant la période là, les femmes ne refusent pas les hommes parce que, elles aussi elles doivent aller semer... les hommes qui sont mariés n'ont pas de problèmes, ce sont les célibataires qui sont obligés de se débrouiller n'importe où.

Le fait d'entretenir des relations sexuelles est supposé augmenter les chances de productivité ou de gain des partenaires sexuelles. Ainsi un homme qui va à la pêche après avoir eu des rapports sexuels avec une femme a d'énormes chances de faire une partie de pêche plus fructueuse qu'un autre qui n'a pas eu de rapport sexuel. En outre, un homme ou une femme qui va semer les grains d'arachide, de mil ou de boutures de manioc et d'ignames sans avoir de relations sexuelles avec un partenaire de sexe opposé, se retrouvera avec une maigre récolte.

Reproduction et sexualité thérapeutique

La sexualité thérapeutique n'est pas une pratique normative dans les communautés ethniques concernées par cette étude. Cependant, elle est une pratique courante. En effet, les guérisseurs traditionnels spécialisés dans l'ethno-gynécologie entretiennent très souvent des relations sexuelles avec les femmes à la recherche d'une grossesse, voir d'un enfant.

Ces relations sexuelles font partie du processus de guérison ou de délivrance des maladies et d'esprits maléfiques à l'origine du mal dont souffre la patiente. Les relations sexuelles entre les tradipraticiens et les femmes de tous les statuts matrimoniaux se caractérisent par l'absence de l'utilisation des préservatifs. Ces rapports sexuels permettent à la femme inféconde ou stérile par exemple, de retrouver sa fécondité ou sa fertilité, d'avoir un enfant (ce sont les cas les plus répandus).

Nous n'avons identifié dans l'ensemble que des aspects négatifs, en ce qui concerne la sexualité rituelle et thérapeutique au sein des groupes ethniques étudiés. Ainsi, au niveau de la sexualité rituelle, les relations sexuelles avec des partenaires inconnues ou différentes des épouses légitimes sont l'expression de l'infidélité, du multi-parténariat sexuel, et des relations sexuelles extra-maritales. Les risques d'infections sont très élevés dans un tel contexte. S'agissant de l'aspect thérapeutique, la négativité de la pratique se traduit par le fait que plusieurs femmes d'horizons diverses se rendent chez le même tradipraticien ou guérisseur avec qui elles ont des relations sexuelles pour trouver la solution à leurs problèmes. L'infection du tradipraticien implique la contamination de toutes ses clientes par voie sexuelle.

Ainsi, les mœurs sexuelles au même titre que les traditions, varient d'une société à l'autre, surtout lorsqu'il s'agit d'analyser les facteurs de permissivité et de non- permissivité (Rwenge 2000). En effet, pour le cas des sociétés permissives, il existe par exemple des cultures où, en cas d'absence prolongée de l'époux, la femme est autorisée à avoir des rapports sexuels extraconjugaux avec un homme faisant partie du lignage de son mari (le cas des Massaï au Nord du Kenya). Ces mœurs sexuelles dans un monde de nomades sont de nature à accroître les risques de vulnérabilité de la femme, même si la finalité est moins le partage des épouses que l'assurance d'une conservation des capacités procréatrices des femmes (Rwenge 2002:24). Dans certains groupes ethniques en Ouganda, des rites funéraires sont pratiqués sur la femme lors du décès de son mari. Il s'agit pour la veuve de se livrer au cours de la nuit d'enterrement à des rapports sexuels avec le frère cadet de son défunt mari pour « chasser », voire exorciser le fantôme de ce dernier (Ilinigumugabo 1989).

Au Cameroun, il existe aussi des mœurs sexuelles qui rendent vulnérable la femme à la maladie. En effet, le cas de la femme Béti dans la société traditionnelle permet de se rendre compte non seulement de la liberté sexuelle qui a toujours été la sienne, mais également de la forme de gestion et de contrôle qu'exerce le conjoint sur sa sexualité (Alexandre et Binet 1958:81 ; Yana 1995:56). Car, si les rapports sexuels sont plus ou moins proscrits aux adolescentes impubères, les jeunes filles célibataires bénéficient quant à elles d'une grande liberté sexuelle tant il est vrai que très peu d'importance est accordée à leur virginité. C'est ainsi que les cas de naissances enregistrés avant le mariage de la jeune fille étaient attendus et présentés comme preuve de sa fertilité (Alexandre et Binet, op. cit., p. 96). Lorsque celle-ci se retrouve dans son foyer, les relations extraconjugales, sans être encouragées, étaient tolérées par le mari cocu.

À ce titre, il n'était pas rare de voir un homme livrer l'une de ses femmes à une forme de « prostitution hospitalière » (Rwenge 2002:37) pour son propre prestige. Il pouvait de ce fait la céder pour une nuit à un ami dont il veut témoigner le grand attachement ou simplement la placer au centre d'un réseau d'échange (Ombolo 1990).

Par contre, dans les sociétés où ces mœurs sexuelles ne sont pas permises comme ce fut le cas dans les sociétés au pouvoir centralisé, la sexualité de la jeune fille était très contrôlée à telle enseigne qu'une grossesse prémaritale ou simplement des relations extraconjugales étaient sévèrement punies. Certaines relations adultérines donnaient lieu à des exclusions de la communauté ou à une élimination physique du coupable, surtout s'il s'agissait d'un « bien » appartenant à un dignitaire traditionnel (Hurault 1962:48-52). Les mutations sociales observées par les effets de l'urbanisation ont conduit néanmoins à l'adoption d'attitudes plus libérales, permissives.

Le lévirat

Le lévirat (« a yekla yik manyan » en langue Basa'a) et (« Ndongou-Réwbé » en « fulfulde ») est une pratique culturelle que l'on retrouve au sein de tous les groupes ethniques étudiés à Lagdo et à Eséka. Cette pratique veut qu'une veuve consente à épouser le frère de son défunt mari. C'est le fait pour l'homme d'hériter de la femme de son frère qui est décédé (APAC–Cameroun, 2004) :

> Chez nous quand un homme meurt, sa femme ne rentre pas dans son village ou sa famille. Elle devient la femme du frère de son mari avec tous ses enfants et biens laissés par son mari. C'est pour ça qu'on donne la dot. Elle doit continuer à faire les enfants avec le frère de son mari, le nom de son mari ne doit pas s'éteindre. On oblige même le frère du mari qui est mort d'épouser cette femme sauf si elle est déjà vieille et qu'elle ne peut plus accoucher (homme de 45 ans, 10-3-2003, Eséka).

Une autre pratique voisine du lévirat est le sororat. C'est une pratique culturelle consistant à remplacer dans un foyer une femme décédée par sa sœur célibataire. Le sororat reste cependant une pratique très peu répandue au sein des différents groupes ethniques à l'exception des Mousgoum.

Le nombre de décès liés au VIH/SIDA au sein des différents groupes ethniques étudiés a une influence encore mitigée que l'on retrouve parmi les groupes de populations ayant un niveau d'éducation au-delà du primaire. Cette couche de la population est sensée être exposée et perméable aux campagnes de sensibilisation sur le VIH/SIDA. C'est ainsi que de plus en plus ils exigent la réalisation du test de séropositivité qui reste néanmoins essentiellement orienté vers la veuve. Mais en zones rurales et au sein de la population n'ayant aucun niveau d'éducation, les comportements à l'égard du lévirat n'ont pas du tout changé. L'acceptation de la pratique conduit au sein des communautés concernées à une intensification des rapports sexuels non protégés ; ce qui accroît les risques de contamination liés au statut sérologique du défunt époux. La pratique des tests de dépistage n'étant pas répandue dans la communauté, les populations sont bien évidemment exposées à l'infection.

La polygamie

Dans toutes les sociétés, les hommes semblent jouir d'une plus grande liberté sexuelle que les femmes. Ce qui leur permet de transgresser, même au sein des groupes christianisés, l'interdit des relations prénuptiales. Si la pratique du mariage est une réalité universelle, le type d'union basé sur la polygamie est considéré comme une pratique rurale. Cette dernière est en rapport avec les représentations et attentes de la société vis-à-vis de la femme. De manière générale, les facteurs évoqués visant à justifier la polygamie sont liés le plus souvent à la stérilité de la première femme, aux conflits qui naissent au sein du couple, à l'amélioration du niveau de vie, ou simplement au besoin d'une main-d'œuvre supplémentaire pour les travaux agricoles ou pour la fabrication des produits laitiers.

Force est de constater que la polygamie est une institution observée aussi bien dans les sociétés centralisées de l'Ouest ou du Nord Cameroun que les sociétés à pouvoir diffus du Centre, Sud et Est. Cette pratique culturelle était alors considérée comme la condition normale d'accroître son capital humain et d'asseoir son autorité au sein de la communauté. Un polygame a non seulement le privilège de désirer et de posséder d'autres femmes en plus de la première, mais aussi de remplacer les épouses âgées par des femmes plus jeunes et sexuellement plus attirantes (Tchak 1999:33).

Dans les sociétés à pouvoir diffus, l'autorité du chef se mesure non pas seulement à l'étendue des biens amassés, mais aussi à sa virilité, au nombre de femmes qu'il possède et également au nombre d'enfants considérés comme une richesse, malgré les conditions difficiles de vie et les épidémies qui expliquent un taux de mortalité infantile assez élevé. Principal agent de production et partant d'enrichissement de l'homme, la femme apparaît en outre comme facteur de renforcement du capital politique et symbolique. Au sujet de la situation de la femme dans la société Fang au Sud Cameroun, Georges Balandier (1963:149-150) affirme que :

La femme assure cette postérité qui est pour tout Fang le premier des biens. Par cette dernière, non seulement, il se montre pleinement mâle mais il obtient une véritable promotion sociale : acquérant une influence qui croit dans la mesure où prospère son groupement familial participant à cette couche sociale prééminente.

Dans les sociétés hiérarchisées de l'Ouest du Cameroun, la forme polygamique du mariage confère, après le décès du mari, une position plus valorisante à la mère de l'héritier par rapport à ses co-épouses (Yana 1995:38). Des analyses faites par S. Tchak (1999:29-30) montrent que malgré la critique adressée de nos jours, la fonction sociale de la polygamie ne devrait pas être reléguée au second plan. En effet, en dépit de la fonction économique qu'elle remplit, la polygamie permet aux co-épouses de se partager les tâches domestiques et champêtres. Par exemple, une des co-épouses peut voyager pour un long moment sans que cela ne se ressente au niveau de l'éducation des enfants ou de la sexualité du mari. La polygamie permettait en outre de réguler les naissances et de permettre à la mère d'allaiter son nouveau-né, sans être tenue d'entretenir des rapports sexuels avec son mari. Cet époux pouvant facilement concéder une longue période d'abstinence sexuelle à la femme qui allaite, dans la mesure où il aura toujours à sa disposition une autre femme disponible.

De nos jours, la confusion entre la puissance de l'homme et sa fécondité reste grande dans la mesure où, freiné par son identification à la bourgeoise occidentale, l'homme est soumis soit par ses amis, soit part sa famille à une très forte pression sociale qui l'oblige à manifester autrement sa virilité à travers le mariage de nombreuses femmes. S'il advenait qu'il refuse d'épouser une deuxième femme, il sera poussé à avoir des relations sexuelles extraconjugales et même à entretenir un « deuxième bureau », une «petite amie » avec laquelle il entretient des rapports sexuels et qui est connue de tous, sauf de la femme légale. Cette situation donne lieu dans certains cas à des naissances hors mariage même si ces jeunes femmes, contrairement à la femme restée à la maison, ont droit à la contraception (Coquery-Vidrovitch 1994:336). C'est dire que le recul de la polygamie dans la société camerounaise contemporaine ne signifie pas pour autant que la monogamie est une réalité. En fait, comme le constate Paulette Béat Songué (1986:116),

Il y a une habitude et une conception de la virilité liée à la puissance qui a été conservée au fil des âges. Il nous semble que dans la société contemporaine camerounaise, les hommes sont restés sexuellement polygames, au plus profond d'eux-mêmes.

C'est dire que la liberté prénuptiale dont bénéficient les hommes est un préalable à des comportements sexuels de polygame ; et que le mariage ne change pas radicalement la propension poussée pour le multipartenariat.

La valeur sexuelle de l'enfant

De manière générale, les sociétés au système social patriarcal accordent plus d'importance à l'enfant de sexe masculin qu'à celui de sexe féminin. En effet, le garçon est présenté comme étant le continuateur de la lignée parentale, le garant des biens de la famille, le successeur du chef de famille alors que la fille est appelée à aller en mariage dans un autre clan. À ce titre, la recherche d'une progéniture de sexe masculin peut conduire une femme à multiplier ses naissances surtout que la recherche d'un enfant de sexe masculin peut conduire l'homme à trouver une seconde femme ou simplement à avoir des naissances hors mariage. Certaines jeunes filles mères quant à elles pensent ainsi avoir plus de chance de garder un homme si elles parviennent à lui donner un garçon. Cette considération de la valorisation du sexe masculin s'observe au niveau des représentations faites par l'un et l'autre sexe ainsi que de la forme différentielle d'éducation transmise.

En effet, l'éducation sexuelle différentielle a nécessairement des répercussions sur les représentations que chaque sexe se fait de l'autre au point où très tôt, les adolescents des deux sexes intériorisent les normes de fonctionnement basées sur des rapports inégaux de dominant et de dominé. Ces rapports de force, sans être totalement connus, trouveront leur fondement au niveau des organes génitaux où le pénis symbolise la virilité, la puissance alors que le vagin renvoie à l'effacement, la honte (Laburthe-Tolra 1981). Pour Tchak (1999:27), le fait que les parents répriment sévèrement les envies sexuelles de leurs filles tout en éprouvant de la fierté à voir leurs fils s'intéresser aux femmes traduit la valeur sociale de la sexualité masculine. Cette initiation qui continue jusqu'à la puberté et à l'apparition des premières règles inculquera à cette future femme l'idéologie selon laquelle sa réussite sociale se définit par rapport à sa possibilité de trouver un mari, mais également par sa capacité à générer des revenus. Les enfants grandiront avec cette représentation que le garçon sera plus tard le sexe dominateur, chef de famille, et la fille celle-là qui doit être assistée par l'homme. Dans toutes les sociétés, l'apprentissage du corps se fait au sein des groupes essentiellement homogènes et unisexués. La phase d'initiation qui intervient à la puberté était chez les garçons une cérémonie pleine de signification qui leur permettait d'entrer dans le monde des hommes, celui du pouvoir. L'initiation des fillettes qui commençait nettement plus tôt que celle des garçons était destinée à les instruire de manière précise sur les jeux sexuels, mais aussi les tabous pesant sur les menstruations et les « secrets » de l'enfantement (Coquery-Vidrovitch 1994:313). On leur enseignait comment s'asseoir de manière décente, comment se comporter devant les hommes à qui elles devraient avoir respect et soumission. Il est attendu de la fille gentillesse, soumission, serviabilité, respect de l'autorité masculine.

Les fonctions vitales dont la femme a la charge sont celles de la reproduction, fonction très valorisée dans une société plus soucieuse de capitaliser en êtres humains (et rapports sociaux) qu'en richesses matérielles durables ; celles de l'entretien des hommes, en assumant la plus large part des tâches de production (Balandier 1974:22). Plus précisément, il s'agit d'une « société virile » qui met les femmes à son service. C'est ce souci de contrôler la sexualité de la jeune fille qui est à l'origine des pratiques telles que le mariage précoce et les mutilations génitales féminines.

Mariage précoce et mutilations génitales féminines

Si le mariage dans la plupart des sociétés africaines ne répond pas en tous points à la définition européenne d'un acte légal d'union entre deux conjoints, il ressort tout de même qu'il renvoie à une forme de mariage reconnue socialement, donnant lieu à une cérémonie et à un échange de biens. Dans certaines sociétés, l'importance accordée à la virginité de la jeune fille était telle qu'à l'âge de 10-13 ans, l'adolescente était arrachée des mains de sa mère pour rejoindre de gré ou de force son nouveau foyer.

L'Organisation Mondiale de la Santé estime qu'environ 40 pour cent des femmes africaines subissent des formes différentes de mutilations génitales. Ces formes variées de mutilations de l'organe reproducteur de la femme, quelle que soit la signification symbolique attribuée au rite (différencier plus clairement les deux sexes, éliminer le clitoris qui est un organe « sale » ou « laid », dangereux à même de tuer un bébé à sa naissance si sa tête l'effleure, ou rendre un homme impuissant si sa verge le rencontre chez les Mossi du Burkina-Faso, etc.), ont pour principales raisons le désir masculin de contrôler la sexualité de la jeune fille exposée, à cet effet, à des traumatismes psychiques et physiologiques. Ainsi, des conséquences à long terme peuvent également suivre à l'instar des abcès et kystes, les viginites et salpingites, des difficultés urinaires, des infections à répétition et même une stérilité. Les pratiques culturelles que véhicule une société peuvent permettre d'en savoir un peu plus sur ses comportements et mœurs sexuelles.

Des actions menées aussi bien par les décideurs que par divers organismes tendent de plus en plus à lutter contre les mariages précoces et les mutilations génitales féminines considérés comme pratiques culturelles traumatisantes pour les jeunes filles. Néanmoins, les éléments culturels sus-mentionnés ne peuvent à eux seuls justifier la vulnérabilité des femmes et partant, la propagation continuelle de l'épidémie du VIH/SIDA, tant les mutations sociales ont modifié considérablement les pratiques qu'on pourrait qualifier de « traditionnelles ». Pour F. Eboko (2000:236), l'expansion de la pandémie du SIDA au Cameroun est en rapport direct avec la crise des modes de régulations socioéconomiques qui avaient cours avant la période d'ajustement structurel, qui a eu pour effet immédiat le glissement d'une majorité de la population dans la pauvreté.

Au sein des groupes ethniques concernés par la pratique de l'excision au Cameroun, la majorité des femmes excisées restent favorables à la continuité de la pratique (par souci de préservation de la coutume) contre une proportion plus grande des jeunes filles adolescentes excisées qui dénoncent cette pratique au motif que leur consentement n'avait pas été requis. Même si l'acceptation de l'excision augmente le niveau d'intégration sociale des filles dans ces communautés, il n'en reste pas moins que cette pratique expose les victimes aux risques d'infection au VIH/SIDA. Par exemple, chez les Kotoko du Nord Cameroun où la pratique est collective, le même instrument (un couteau bien tranchant et plus récemment la lame de rasoir), est utilisé pour toutes les filles soumises à l'opération les unes après les autres. L'infection au VIH/SIDA de la première fille ou de la deuxième fille à être excisée peut entraîner la contamination à travers l'instrument utilisé.

Scarifications corporelles

La scarification corporelle désignée sous le terme de « Njehel «chez les Bassa, et « Yiérol » ou « Toupago » chez les Foulbé et les Mafa est une pratique culturelle qui a lieu sous diverses formes et est soutenue par autant d'idéologies. Chez les Mafa et les Guiziga, elle a une fonction socialisatrice, parce qu'elle représente une identité ethnique et culturelle (Balafres). La scarification chez les Foulbé, les Guiziga et les Toupouri a une fonction esthétique (perforation des lèvres ou des narines : perforation simple des lèvres). Enfin, au sein de tous les groupes ethniques étudiés elle a une fonction thérapeutique (blessure de la peau).

Chaque type de scarification constitue une pratique particulière ayant une idéologie précise. S'agissant de la dimension identitaire de la scarification, on retrouve les balafres chez les Guiziga et les Mafa de sexe masculin. Cette pratique consiste à faire des traits le long des joues gauche et droite, généralement trois traits de chaque côté. La pratique a lieu de manière individuelle mais aussi collective. En ce qui concerne le type collectif, des jeunes enfants et parfois des adolescents de la même génération sont regroupés pour subir la pratique qui est effectuée par le spécialiste de la localité à l'aide d'une lamelle de tige de mil ou de couteau. Les blessures occasionnées, dans lesquelles est appliquée une poudre cicatrisante doivent rester entrouvertes jusqu'à la guérison ; afin de mieux faire ressortir la fente. Les garçons passent en fait les uns après les autres sous le couteau du praticien. Les balafres participeront ainsi de leur beauté et feront d'eux de vrais hommes Guiziga ou Mafa.

S'agissant de l'aspect esthétique, les jeunes filles foulbé (imitées de plus par les autres groupes ethniques du Lagdo) utilisent des épines ou des aiguilles pour se perforer légèrement toutes les lèvres supérieures et inférieures. Elles appliquent sur les lèvres ensanglantées un liquide noir tiré de l'écorce d'un arbre (mais aujourd'hui les filles utilisent de plus en plus un produit appelé black qui sert à noircir les cheveux) pour les rendre plus noires.

> On fait ça avec les épines. On pique d'abord, on pique, on pique tes lèvres là jusqu'à le sang coule. Quand le sang cesse de couler, l'eau commence à sortir alors, et puis on met le black. On utilise douze épines pour une personne, si c'est encore bon, ton amie peut encore faire sa part avec. Ce sont les épines de jujubes (Aminata, 18 ans habitant de Lagdo).

La couleur noire irréversible que prennent désormais les lèvres participe de leur beauté et de leur charme. D'une manière générale, elles le font les unes les autres avec les mêmes foins d'épines ou d'aiguilles.

La troisième forme de scarification qui a une fonction thérapeutique concerne tous les groupes ethniques étudiés.

> Quand tu es malade, tu vas à l'hôpital, on ne peut pas te soigner, on part seulement chez le marabout, il te blesse avec la lame qui est toujours à côté de lui et il met le produit. Tu guéris même si c'est un sorcier qui te cherche. On fait aussi çà pour te protéger contre les mauvais esprits et les sorciers (une femme, de Lagdo).

Cette forme est en générale pratiquée par les guérisseurs traditionnels qui blessent légèrement la peau de leurs patients à l'aide d'un couteau ou d'une lame de rasoir. Malgré le caractère individuel de la pratique, il convient de relever le fait que l'outil (lame de rasoir ou couteau) utilisé par le guérisseur est soigneusement gardé par ce dernier pour une utilisation ultérieure sur un autre client. La pratique vise à prévenir contre les maladies et malheurs futurs ou ceux dont souffre le patient. À l'intérieur de la blessure faite à l'épaule, au poignet, sur le dos ou sur le front, le tradipraticien introduit généralement une poudre dont lui seul connaît la nature et parfois les vertus.

Les scarifications corporelles sont apparues au courant de toute notre étude comme un facteur ne pouvant que favoriser la propagation du VIH/SIDA. Nous constatons que dans toutes les formes, il y a effusion de sang et utilisation d'un seul outil pour tous les individus. Les outils imbibés du sang d'une première personne sont utilisés immédiatement pour une deuxième, ainsi de suite. Le virus peut ainsi se transmettre facilement d'une personne à une autre et se répandre dans les différentes communautés. En général, les réactions concernant premièrement les scarifications ayant une fonction thérapeutique se caractérisent essentiellement par l'acceptation, car il s'agit d'une pratique culturelle faisant partie de l'ethnomédecine, du système thérapeutique des groupes ethniques étudiés (cf. APAC–Cameroun 2004).

Facteurs socio-économiques, mutations sociales et modèles de comportements sexuels

Les comportements sexuels des jeunes et adolescents au Cameroun restent liés à l'évolution de la société globale, au contexte de changement rapide que connaît cette société. Cette situation entraîne nécessairement des incidences sur la propagation du VIH/SIDA et la prise en charge des malades. Pour Béat Songué (1998:177), ces changements sont la cause de l'introduction des valeurs et modèles étrangers en matière de sexualité (mariages, rôle de la cellule familiale, modalités du rapport sexuel, etc.), mais aussi de l'évolution du niveau de l'éducation, de la formation, des infrastructures sanitaires publiques et privées, et de l'emploi. A ce titre, les conduites qui se reproduisent dans les choix, les attitudes et comportements individuels des jeunes et adolescents dans un milieu social donné leur seront dictées par les valeurs véhiculées dans le groupe d'appartenance.

Propagation du VIH/SIDA et impuissance de l'État

Une certaine grille de lecture permet d'établir une corrélation entre la progression rapide de la pandémie du SIDA, l'engagement de l'Etat dans la lutte contre ce fléau et la situation de désarroi dans laquelle vivent la plupart des Camerounais suite aux mesures internationales d'Ajustement structurel des économies des pays africains. En effet, avant la mise sous tutelle de l'économie camerounaise par les institutions de Bretton Woods au début des années 1990, c'est à l'État que revenait le rôle de régulateur social et politique par sa capacité de distribution des revenus, de contrôle du jeu politique et de promotion des valeurs idéologiques qui en font un véritable moteur des aspirations de mobilité sociale et des représentations sociales qui confortent l'illusion de sa toute puissance. La mise sur pied des Programmes d'ajustements structurels ne fit qu'accroître le nombre de populations misérables, notamment en milieu urbain. Un rapport de la Banque mondiale publié en décembre 1995 estimait le pourcentage des familles vivant en dessous du seuil de pauvreté à 20 pour cent à Yaoundé et à 30 pour cent à Douala. A cette crise économique s'est ajoutée une crise politique qui pour certains analystes, annonçait le désarroi d'un État en voie de privatisation. Face à ce désengagement de l'État de plusieurs de ses fonctions régaliennes, les mesures qui tenaient lieu de politique gouvernementale de lutte contre le SIDA au Cameroun ne partaient pas d'une réelle volonté de la part des décideurs. Pour F. Eboko (2000:237),

> L'inféodation du Programme national de lutte contre le sida (PNLS), dès 1987, aux financements de bailleurs de fonds étrangers, le contenu ambigü de la communication sociale relative à la prévention, la faiblesse manifeste de la volonté politique en face des questions liées à la sexualité et le refuge dans des réponses scientifico-techniques montrent les limites de l'État camerounais dans sa gestion des risques relatifs au VIH/sida.

À ce titre, la propagation du virus du SIDA est à attribuer aussi bien au changement social global qui affecte de manière radicale la société camerounaise, qu'aux pratiques sociales anciennes. En effet, si les rapports sexuels avant le mariage étaient considérés comme indécents pour la famille de la jeune fille, la femme mariée par contre semblait avoir acquis le droit à l'usage de son corps. En pays Bassa par exemple, V. Coquery-Vidrovitch (1994:189) observe qu'en cas d'adultère, l'amant se devait de donner au mari cocu un poulet, ce qui permettait d'officialiser la liaison tout en reconnaissant le préjudice causé par cette polyandrie tacite. Le changement observé dans différentes cultures, conséquence de l'urbanisation et de la croissance démographique, a entraîné nécessairement une modification des mœurs sexuelles et une gestion plus individuelle que communautaire de la sexualité de la jeune fille. Ces facteurs sont générés soit par la pression démographique, soit par les conditions socio-économiques précaires des personnes appartenant à certaines couches de la population.

Poussée de la fécondité et incidence du VIH/SIDA

Différentes études ont pu montrer que l'Afrique au sud du Sahara détient le taux de fécondité le plus élevé du monde (Tabutin 1988). Pour ce qui est du Cameroun, des Enquêtes démographiques et de Santé montrent que la fécondité demeure élevée avec en moyenne 5 enfants par femme, avec cependant une fécondité précoce élevée dans la tranche d'âge se situant entre 15 et 19 ans, soit 142 pour mille. Celle-ci augmentera rapidement pour atteindre des maxima dans la tranche 20-24 ans, soit 273 pour mille et entre 25-29 ans, soit 244 pour mille. Cette poussée de la fécondité se maintient longtemps dans les tranches d'âges de 30 à 34 ans, soit 189 pour mille et de 35 à 39 ans, soit 136 pour mille. Par la suite, ce taux va décroître très rapidement.

En outre, la même étude révèle que le niveau de fécondité est plus fort en milieu rural qu'en milieu urbain tant il est vrai que l'indice synthétique de fécondité est de 3,1 dans les villes de Yaoundé et Douala, 4,5 dans les autres villes, mais se situe à 5,8 en milieu rural. La relative constante des niveaux actuels de fécondité permet d'estimer le nombre d'enfants d'une femme en zone rurale à 2,7 enfants de plus qu'une femme de Yaoundé et Douala et à 1,3 enfants de plus qu'une femme des autres villes. Toutefois, quelque soit leur milieu de résidence, les femmes réalisent le maximum de leur fécondité entre 25 et 29 ans. Cette pression démographique observée découle non seulement de la représentation que l'Africain se fait de la famille, mais aussi des comportements actuels en matière de sexualité. A ce titre, l'enfant en milieu africain continue d'être perçu à la fois comme une valeur biologique et culturelle. L. Roussel (1995:140) note à ce titre que « la famille est le lieu obligé de cette double survie puisqu'elle assure à la fois le renouvellement des générations et par l'éducation, la permanence des valeurs sociétales ».

Cette importance accordée à la fécondité de la femme est de nature à rendre fragile la santé de reproduction de la mère et même à la rendre vulnérable aux IST dont le SIDA. Comment peut-il en être autrement quand on sait par exemple qu'en Afrique, le nombre de naissances, surtout les garçons, détermine le statut social de celle-ci (Akam 1999 et Rwenge 2000). C'est ce qui explique que la fécondité élevée est un trait caractéristique et reluisant de l'image de la femme. À ce titre, plus une femme est féconde, plus grand sera son statut au sein de la société, et toute remise en question de cette fonction maternelle de la femme peut conduire cette dernière à la marginalisation (Dozon et Guillaume 1994:179-223) et au mépris.

En replaçant la fécondité dans son système culturel, l'on constate aisément que les attitudes des personnes sont révélatrices des rapports et des comportements les plus fondamentaux de l'homme et de la femme. À ce titre, l'amélioration du statut de la femme passe nécessairement par une action sur la fécondité, les conditions de vie et de santé tant en milieu urbain qu'en zone rurale.

Facteurs socioéconomiques et démographiques

La capacité de la famille et de la collectivité à prendre soin des malades du SIDA reste tributaire dans une grande mesure du niveau de revenus et des réseaux sociaux. Or, la crise économique et la paupérisation qui touchent les populations depuis plus d'une décennie ont permis de développer des nouvelles stratégies de riposte à la crise, et la sexualité en est une pour bon nombre. C'est ainsi que dans les grandes agglomérations s'est développée une sexualité de crise (Eboko 2000:245-246) où, en plus des prostituées habituelles, se sont ajoutées des prostituées occasionnelles (dont les charmes sont monnayés ponctuellement), les jeunes femmes qui combinent leurs aspirations affectives aux besoins matériels pour une polyandrie plus ou moins officieuse (un « sponsor » qui finance et le « meilleur petit » pour le recours affectif) et enfin les « filles à marier » dont les espoirs familiaux et personnels sont exclusivement portés vers la recherche d'un bon partenaire pour la vie.

Le plus souvent, les personnes qui décèdent sont généralement ceux sur qui reposent tous les espoirs de la famille tant il est vrai que l'épidémie décime le groupe d'âge le plus actif et le plus productif (20-25 ans). Des études ont montré que la disparition d'un membre de la famille adulte dans la force de l'âge a des répercussions à long terme sur le reste de la famille. Dans cet ordre d'idées, c'est la femme qui prend soin du mari malade jusqu'à sa mort. Lorsque le cas inverse se produit par contre, la femme est ramenée soit chez sa mère, soit auprès de ses sœurs ou de ses filles. Lorsque la femme survit à son mari, elle devient entièrement responsable de la famille, ce qui l'amène à se remarier ou à se livrer à la prostitution, pour la survie de ses enfants.

L'âge du premier rapport sexuel a considérablement reculé à cause d'un ensemble de facteurs : l'urbanisation rapide et la scolarisation de plus en plus tardive des jeunes filles, le travail des femmes ainsi que de nouveaux modèles de vie que véhiculent les médias occidentaux. Le changement observé concerne plus les circonstances de ces premiers rapports sexuels. Avant, la coutume voulait que la jeune fille soit placée sous la surveillance et la protection d'une tante paternelle avant ses premières règles. De nos jours, il y a moins de surveillance et les rapports sexuels avant le mariage ne sont pratiquement plus sanctionnés.

Le phénomène migratoire et l'incidence sur la santé de la famille

Le déplacement des populations d'une région à une autre est un phénomène social ancien qui concerne à la fois riches et pauvres, jeunes et vieux, mariés et célibataires, divorcés et veufs. Les raisons évoquées visant à justifier ces migrations sont diverses et complexes. Ce sont : de la recherche d'un emploi ou d'une vie meilleure, la fuite de la guerre, la poursuite des études, le rejet par les autres membres de la communauté et bien d'autres causes encore. Cette recherche d'une vie meilleure conduit le plus souvent les personnes démunies à entretenir des relations sexuelles avec des personnes plus âgées moins pour le plaisir que pour de l'argent. En effet, l'expression sexe pour de l'argent renvoie à cette pratique répandue qui consiste à monnayer les relations sexuelles. Cette expression est également utilisée pour désigner les filles ou les femmes qui ont plusieurs partenaires, même s'il n'y a pas échange d'argent tandis que la prostituée est cette femme qui entretient des rapports sexuels en dehors du mariage. Une étude menée en Ouganda a montré qu'un pourcentage assez élevé de veufs âgés de 30 à 40 ans et de veuves de 15 à 44 ans quittent leur domicile conjugal. Les jeunes veuves quant à elles retournent auprès de leurs parents. La connaissance de cette pandémie a considérablement réduit le taux de migrants stigmatisés par le SIDA. En outre, les veufs possédant des enfants sont plus enclins à la migration que ceux qui n'en possèdent pas. Cette trajectoire migratoire peut être relié au SIDA dans la mesure où la maladie a permis aux veuves d'hériter des biens ou de se remarier. Plusieurs d'entre elles sont expulsées du village et voient leurs biens saisis. Pour échapper ainsi à la stigmatisation sociale, beaucoup quittent la région pour s'occuper de leur famille. Les veufs âgés de 29 ans et les veuves de 30 ans et plus constituent la catégorie sociale qui émigre le plus. Les plus âgées vont retrouver leur fils ou parents puisqu'elles ont moins de chance de se retrouver à nouveau sous un toit conjugal.

Famille et prise en charge des personnes vivant avec le VIH/SIDA

L'image véhiculée sur le SIDA, du fait même de l'absence de remèdes et de traitement efficace contre la maladie, a influencé dans une grande mesure les réseaux communautaires de prise en charge des malades. Cette prise en charge reste fonction de l'ethos social ancré dans les représentations populaires de la maladie au Cameroun. Ainsi, des stéréotypes ont été véhiculés à propos du VIH/SIDA présenté comme étant « la maladie de la honte », symbole du « relâchement des mœurs », résultat du « vagabondage sexuel » et de tout un ensemble de propos comportementalistes qui conduisent à culpabiliser moins ceux qui continuent d'entretenir des relations sexuelles conformes aux normes et à la morale que ces couches de la population identifiées très tôt comme groupes à risque (jeunes scolaires et universitaires, militaires, prostituées, transporteurs). En matière de prise en charge, le choix de la personne appelée à s'occuper d'un malade de SIDA dépend d'un certain nombre de facteurs qui vont de la perception que l'on a de la maladie, du niveau de revenus de la personne et de sa famille, de sa situation matrimoniale, de la gravité de son état de santé ou encore celle de son conjoint. Au sein d'un couple, les deux partenaires s'occupent mutuellement l'un de l'autre. Les célibataires quant à eux sont généralement pris en charge par leur mère lorsqu'elle est vivante, leurs frères ou sœurs dans le cas contraire.

Conclusion

Cette étude montre que l'élément culturel est un facteur non négligeable si l'on veut engager une action efficace de lutte contre une épidémie comme celle du VIH/SIDA. Toutefois, les facteurs culturels ne suffisent pas à expliquer entièrement l'ampleur et la propagation du VIH/SIDA dans la mesure où les questions de sexualité et de santé de la reproduction se posent avec acuité. La pression des valeurs nouvelles fait en sorte que les jeunes générations ne parviennent pas à résister à l'attrait de la modernité et par conséquent, à reproduire les schèmes comportementaux transmis par les parents. Cette situation peut être observée par exemple au niveau du choix des partenaires sexuels pour une liaison temporaire ou pour la vie de couple.

Il serait intéressant d'initier des études anthropologiques spécifiques sur l'origine des comportements sexuels pour mieux comprendre l'effet des valeurs culturelles sur la propagation et le traitement du VIH/SIDA, avec un accent particulier sur les groupes présentés comme étant les plus vulnérables (jeunes adolescents, prostituées, militaires, femmes libres, camionneurs, enfants des rues, etc.). En outre, l'analyse de la relation existante entre le taux de prévalence du VIH et la pauvreté, l'évaluation de l'effet des valeurs culturelles sur le VIH/SIDA, la détermination de l'influence du changement d'attitudes à l'égard des traditions sur les différents aspects de la propagation, du traitement et de la prise en charge de la maladie se présentent comme autant de domaines qui peuvent permettre de mieux comprendre la corrélation qui existe entre la propagation de la maladie et les facteurs socioculturels au Cameroun.

Bibliographie

Akam E., 1999, « Infécondité et sous-fécondité : évaluation et recherche de facteurs — le cas du Cameroun », in *Les Cahiers de l'IFORD*, no. 26, IFORD, Yaoundé, octobre.

Alexandre P., Binet, J., 1958, *Le groupe dit Pahouin Fang*, Boulou, Beti, Paris, PUF.

Andezian S., 1985, « Nouvelles représentations de la santé et de la maladie : la dialectique entre traditions et modernité », Université de Laval.

APAC-Cameroun, 1994, « Étude de base communautaire sur les facteurs socioculturels de la propagation et de la prévention du VIH/SIDA au Cameroun ». Rapport de recherche.

Balandier G., 1974, *Anthropologiques*, Paris, PUF.

Balandier G., 1963, *Sociologie actuelle de l'Afrique noire*, Paris, PUF (2e éd.)

Beat Songue P., 1998, « Influence du milieu social sur la sexualité et les comportements reproducteurs des adolescents au Sud Cameroun », in Kuate-Defo, B. (dir.), *Sexualité reproductive durant l'adolescence en Afrique. Avec une attention particulière sur le Cameroun*, Québec, EDICONSEIL Inc.

Beat Songue P., 1986, *La prostitution en Afrique, l'exemple de Yaoundé*, Paris, L'Harmattan, 154 p.

Beker ch., Dozon j.p., Obbo ch. & Touré M. (Eds.), 1999, *Vivre et penser le sida en Afrique*, CODESRIA-Karthala-IRD.

Caldwell J. C. & al., 1989, « The Social Context of AIDS in Sub-Saharan Africa », *Population and Development Review*, no. 15, p.185-234.

Caldwell J. C., 1993, «Tenth Transition: The Cultural Social and Behavioural Determinants of Health in the Third World », *Social Science and Medicine*, Vol. 36, no. 2.

Care International, 2001, *Analyse de la situation du VIH/SIDA sur les axes routiers du Cameroun*, Yaoundé.

Clumeck N., 1989, *Heterosexual-promiscuity Among African Patient with AIDS*, N. Eng. J. Med.

CNLS, 2001, *Guide technique pour la prévention de la transmission mère-enfant du VIH au Cameroun*, Yaoundé : Imprimerie Saint Paul.

Coquery-Vidrovitch C., 1994, *Les africaines* (Histoire des femmes d'Afrique noire du XIXe au XXe siècle), Paris, Éd. Desjonquères.

Dozon J. P. et Guillaume A.,1994, « Contextes, conséquences socio-économiques et coûts du sida », *Populations africaines et Sida*, Paris, La Découverte / CEPED, p. 179-223.

Eboko F., 2000, « Risque-sida, sexualité et pouvoirs. La puissance de l'État en question » in Courade, G. (dir.), *Le désarroi camerounais : l'épreuve de l'économie-monde*, Paris, Karthala, pp. 235-262.

Hurault J., 1962, *La structure sociale des Bamiléké*, La Haye, Mouton.

Ilinigumugabo A., 1989, *L'espacement des naissances au Rwanda : niveau, causes et conséquences*, Louvain-La-Neuve, CIACO/Institut de démographie, 243 p.

Kimani, V., 1989, *Sexuality in Africa: The Role of Cultural Belief and Behaviour in the Control of AIDS*, Montreal.

Laburthe-Tolra P., 1981, *Les seigneurs de la forêt. Essai sur le passé historique, l'organisation sociale et les normes ethniques des anciens Béti du Sud Cameroun*, Paris : Sorbonne.

Nebout N., 1994, *Lumières sur le SIDA, Les classiques africains*, Versailles, 103 p.

Ombolo J. P., 1990, *Sexe et société en Afrique noire*, Paris, L'Harmattan.

ONUSIDA, 2000, *Le SIDA en Afrique : pays par pays*, Genève.

ONUSIDA/UNESCO, 1999, « L'approche culturelle de la prévention et du traitement du VIH/SIDA, l'expérience de l'Ouganda » − Rapport national.

Rosenheim M. et al., 1989, *SIDA : Infection à VIH. Aspects en zone tropicale*, Paris, AUPELF/ELLIPSES.

Roussel L., 1995, « Fécondité et famille » in Gérard, H. et Piché, V. (dir.) *La sociologie des populations*, Montréal : PUM ; Paris : AUPELF/UREF.

Rwenge M., 1999, « Changement social, structures familiales et fécondité en Afrique subsaharienne : le cas du Cameroun », in *Les Cahiers de l'IFORD*, no. 26, IFORD, Yaoundé, octobre.

Rwenge M., 1999, *Facteurs contextuels des comportements sexuels (le cas des jeunes de la ville de Bamenda, Cameroun)*, UEPA/IFORD, no. 40, 164 p.

Rwenge M., 2002, « Culture, genre, comportements sexuels et MST/SIDA au Cameroun », IFORD, *Les Cahiers de l'IFORD*, no. 28, 276 p.

Sabatier R., 1989, *L'épidémie raciste*, Paris, l'Harmattan, Institut Panos.

Tabutin. D., 1988, *Population et sociétés en Afrique noire*, Paris, L'Harmattan.

Tchak S., 1999, *La sexualité féminine en Afrique : domination masculine et libération féminine*, Paris, L'Harmattan.

Touré, M., 1995, « À propos des facteurs anthropologiques de la propagation du SIDA en Afrique », *Anthropologie africaine*, Revue de l'Association panafricaine d'Anthropologie, vol. II, n°2, pp.129-143.

Yana, D., 1995, « À la recherche des modèles culturels de la fécondité : une étude exploratoire auprès de Bamiléké et Béti de la ville et de la campagne », Institut de démographie de l'UCL, Louvain-La-Neuve, Académia, Paris, L'Harmattan.